# TRAVELING

## ...LIKE EVERYBODY ELSE

### A PRACTICAL GUIDE FOR DISABLED TRAVELERS

Jacqueline Freedman

Susan Gersten

## ADAMA BOOKS

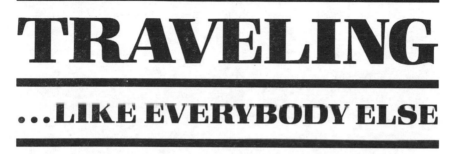

Copyright © 1987 Jacqueline Freedman and Susan Gersten
All rights reserved

Library of Congress Cataloging-in-Publication Data
Freedman, Jacqueline.
    Traveling—like everybody else.

    Includes index.
    1. Physically handicapped—Travel.   I. Gersten,
Susan.   II. Title.
HV3022.F74   1987   910.2'02'0240816       87–1811
ISBN 0–915361–77–9 (pbk.)

Book Design by Irwin Rosenhouse

ADAMA BOOKS, 306 West 38 Street, New York, N.Y. 10018

Printed in Israel

**To Michael and David:**
*For your independence, for working so hard to excel, and for your willingness to push the wheelchair—whether to the lingerie department at Harrod's, the grocery store in St. Moritz or to the top of the Acropolis in Athens. Thank you for sharing your lives with me.*

**To Karl:**
*For his compassion, patience, sensitivity, and great pride in me. Thank you for supporting my efforts, my dreams and my very soul.*

S.G.


**My gratitude to Irv, Michele, Elaine and Amy**
*for their encouragement, love and belief that this book would come to fruition. Their understanding during the many hours I spent with my typewriter is greatly appreciated.*
*My thanks to Gail whose editing and insistence on verbal clarity made this book a reality.*

J. F.

# CONTENTS

# YOU CAN TRAVEL

Who says disabled people can't travel? Of course you can. Whether you are blind, have a disabling disease, are a paraplegic, have cancer, or suffer from one of the multitude of other disablers, you certainly can travel. Disabled doesn't mean unable. It merely means that you have to plan more carefully and be better organized, which isn't new since you always have to pursue your daily activities in a carefully planned manner. It is essential that you not allow your disability to imprison you. Give yourself the opportunity to grow. Feel free. Will you be tired? Yes. Will you wonder what on earth you are doing away from home? No! When you travel, you will be enjoying the pleasures of exciting new places or revisiting places you may have been years ago. As a disabled person myself, I can tell you that the thrill will be greater than that which other visitors experience because life's obstacles teach us to enjoy life's pleasures more.

Although there are 36 million disabled people in the United States, only one in six was born that way. Why shouldn't you continue—or, better yet, begin—to see the world? Historical, recreational and cultural events are there for the taking. Of course, there are problems such as inaccessible buildings, uncut curbs, and parking lots without spaces marked for the handicapped, but as more disabled people are integrated into the community, barriers are slowly beginning to disappear. Don't be discouraged. You can and should avail yourself of the opportunities that exist throughout the world. This book is written to assist you with all aspects of your trip so that you may take advantage of these travel opportunities.

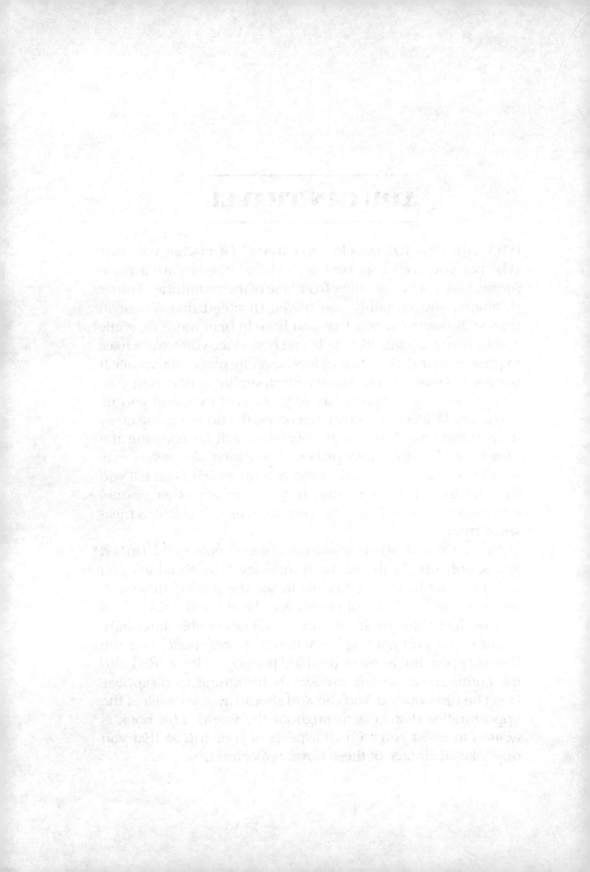

# WHAT, ME TRAVEL?

*Can I Go?* How can I go? It's so expensive. I may get caught in another country and find that I need a doctor. How will I know what doors my wheelchair will fit through? What will foreign people think of me? I can barely get around at home; how on earth will I manage in a foreign land?

It is natural to doubt whether you can travel. Activities aren't easy for us. If you are informed and realistic, most questions can be solved, but guilt and fear are our biggest enemies. Why should I spend the money if I can't be active the entire day? Isn't it decadent to spend money to nap in London when I could be doing the same thing at home?

Our illnesses may cost a lot of money, but that doesn't mean we aren't also entitled to pleasure. There is no reason to feel guilty about lying down for half a day, if, realistically, that means you feel well enough to pursue your journey.

Traveling builds confidence in your capabilities as you learn that you are able to overcome difficult circumstances. The ability to travel severs the bonds of disability. As the disabled learn this, their voices are being heard more and more as they demand services. Airlines and railroads are responding. Although traveling could still be made easier, it is now possible to visit most places. Be the beneficiary of this freedom and independence that only you can fully appreciate.

*You Can Go—Your Way.* Fears can be conquered by information and you need more information than other travelers. There are many different ways to explore the world; choose what is best for you. It is not selfish, but wise, to ensure that plans are conceived according to your priorities, abilities and energy levels. You know your strengths and weaknesses best and your trip must be planned accordingly. If you're tired by midafternoon, set aside time for a nap everyday. It is all right to get tired and rest until you are refreshed enough to pursue your agenda. Many people who are not disabled also find rest essential to traveling. It may be that you are only able to sightsee in the morning and spend the remainder of the day resting. That's okay. Perhaps you can walk with a cane in the morning and use a wheelchair in the afternoon. If so, plan your mornings visiting places inaccessible to wheelchairs and your afternoons on long distance touring more easily accomplished in a wheelchair. If you get tired, rest until you feel well enough to continue your journey.

Each of us has his or her own unique disability level, and different types of pain and needs that require different time schedules. There's no one right way to travel. Do things according to your own capabilities. If you have trouble breathing because of emphysema, you won't want to travel to a small town high in the mountains of Mexico; try visiting the lowlands. People with arthritis would not enjoy a trip during the rainy season, but the dry season would be perfect. If you enjoy the theatre at night, but find that you are exhausted by noon, nap in the afternoon or stay in bed all day so that you can go. If it is important to you, find a way to do it. Bus tours, where you are seated, are less tiring and may prove more enjoyable than touring an endless number of museums, and can provide a taste of the entire country. The joy of tailoring the trip for yourself is that you can make the most of your time and energy.

***Why Wait—You Will Never Be Wealthier or Healthier.*** Using your money to travel is not frivolous. Considering the recreational as well as psychological rewards, it's a bargain. There isn't much point in waiting until you have saved more money, for one thing is certain: the longer you put off spending money the more expensive it will be in the future. Martyrdom went out with Joan of Arc. It isn't wrong to take care of yourself psychologically as well as physically. Like everyone else, you are entitled to pleasure regardless of how much money is spent for your medical bills and special needs. You deserve it. Give yourself a gift that grows in value as memories linger: the adventure will be even more meaningful in the future if you are not feeling well and you can make your day better by recalling the past.

Don't put it off. Start planning today. You aren't in the same situation as the young parents who must defer traveling until their children are older. It's not necessary to postpone life's pleasures for who knows what tomorrow will bring.

Postponing your trip in hopes that you might feel better or stronger in the future isn't very realistic either. If your physical prognosis is uncertain, it is even more essential that you enjoy life now. Grab the opportunity while you can because in a few years you may look back and say, "Why didn't I go when I could? I didn't enjoy myself enough. I wish I had done things differently and not let life pass me by." Fighting depression and defeat through travel can be exhilarating and addictive.

A wheelchair, walker, or crutches mean mobility. They mean not having to stay in the house. They should also mean not having to stay in your own town, city, or country. You can travel . . . like everyone else. The hardest part of traveling is convincing yourself that you can do it. You can! You can!

***I Did It. I Am Here.*** The real success in traveling by wheelchair or other aids is knowing that you are capable of going someplace different. Wheelchair travelers soon discover that the joy in a trip is not the sights you see, the bargains you buy, or the wonderful food you eat, but the ability to say to yourself, "I did it. I am here. My trip may be different from other people's, but I *can* travel." Using a wheelchair or other equipment need not make you a prisoner. Instead, let them open up your world to a more active life. It just takes more planning and know-how.

***Planning in Advance.*** Disabled or not, planning is an essential ingredient of traveling that adds excitement and anticipation to the trip. Since the disabled must plan even more, they get even more enjoyment from this phase of the trip.

After you have decided to make a journey, the most important decision is how you want to travel: in a group or independently. The average travel agency is not familiar with the needs of disabled travelers. Most lack the information essential to your daily living, and the willingness or the time to research special accommodations. Therefore, whether you choose to travel in a group or independently, your local travel agent is probably not your prime source of assistance in planning your trip.

***There are Other Resources Besides Standard Travel Agents.*** There are special experienced travel firms devoted to arranging tours for the disabled by air, ship, bus or train (see list of tour operators who specialize in tours for the disabled, p. *157*). For those who feel more comfortable traveling with other disabled people, or want the services of the doctor or nurse who usually accompanies these trips, there are many group-sponsored tours including specific types, such as for those with multiple sclerosis, arthritis or muscular dystrophy. There is even a cruise designed for patients with kidney problems who need a dialysis machine.

Consult the telephone directory to get the telephone numbers of organizations related to specific disabilities. The people at these organizations can tell you about planned trips or refer you to an appropriate person to aid in your travels.

***Going Alone.*** It is not only possible but quite wonderful to travel independently as it provides the ultimate opportunity for freedom in choosing where to go and with whom. It also allows for adjustment of schedules for individual needs. Without the help of travel specialists, independent travel requires work to provide yourself with necessary information. The extra effort is worthwhile because, in researching your trip, you are not only sure that your needs will be met, but also you will learn a lot about your destination. Planning your trip is one more activity that you can do on your own.

***Do You Need a Traveling Companion?*** Independent travel need not mean traveling alone. Besides, it's more enjoyable to share experiences. But with the disabled, companionship can either be a luxury or a necessity. To make this determination, you must answer the crucial question, "Do I need an aide or companion?" To assess your personal needs, ask yourself the following questions:

Can I handle my own luggage in countries that don't have porters?

Can I lift my luggage onto a baggage rack or the bed in order to unpack?

Can I unpack all my clothes myself?

Can I hang my clothes on hangers and put them away?

Can I use a regular pay phone or must I depend on telephones for the disabled?

Can I reach the counter in most banks to exchange money or cash travelers checks?

Can I rent a car in a foreign country or must I have a special license or a car with special controls?

Can I walk or push my wheelchair over uneven cobblestone streets so prevalent in Europe?

Is my balance good enough to open stuck dresser drawers so common in European hotels?

In Cairo, Egypt, the airport doesn't have porters which means you must carry your own luggage through the airport and lift it on and off racks. In fact, in most airports, airline personnel will only take you to the luggage pick-up point and it is up to you to get your luggage to a car or taxi.

When considering Europe, you must decide whether you can cope with the many cobblestone streets. Walking is precarious, and pushing a wheelchair even more difficult. A wheelchair can easily get caught between the cobblestones, dumping you into the street. An aide could be helpful in this situation. Whether you regularly use a wheelchair or not, you may want to consider renting one while you are traveling over quaint and pretty streets that can be hazardous to any walker.

Aside from physical obstacles, there is the question of the

unexpected—how well can you adjust? An indicator of ability to travel without an aide is your capability of dealing with unexpected situations. Unpleasant surprises are difficult under any circumstances, but much more so if you are traveling without someone to assist you. The last chapter of this book gives advice on what to do when disasters occur.

If you have any doubts at all, travel with someone. It is frightening and dangerous to be in a foreign country and suddenly realize you can't manage because you overestimated your capabilities or because the services you take for granted at home are not available.

***Who Makes a Good Aide?*** If you should decide that you need an aide, it can be anyone from a child to an elderly person as long as he or she is able to handle your wheelchair and assume some responsibility. Children physically capable of assisting are often ideal traveling companions. My twelve-year-old son became a valuable asset when we were traveling in England. He had boundless energy for pushing a wheelchair and for fetching magazines from across the room. At the same time, he exuded enthusiasm because of the new and different world to which he was being exposed. Also, it is often easier to ask a child or teenager to run errands than to ask another adult.

A physically able, retired friend or relative can also be an excellent choice. They may have the time to spare and an unexpected offer to travel could fulfill a long held desire. The elderly, like the disabled, often postpone traveling because of physical or monetary concerns and fear. Some may never have traveled, and your need could be an excuse to turn a dream into a reality. Sharing the pleasure of an enthusiastic companion can be one of the most important ingredients of your trip.

In deciding whom to ask, don't overlook the obvious. In your selection, you should consider how much you enjoy the person's company. It certainly wouldn't be much fun to travel with cranky Uncle Jim, regardless of his availability.

Once you've chosen your companion, involve him or her in planning the trip. Aside from the usual courtesies of accommodations that all fellow travelers must make, it is important for the person to be well aware of the areas in which you require assistance since he or she must be both willing and capable of performing the necessary duties.

If you can't find someone in your immediate circle of friends or relatives, ask them to help you in your search. Perhaps a friend from work, someone in a club you belong to, or even a friend of a friend may want to join you. Your priest, minister or rabbi meets many people and may know someone. Word of mouth is an excellent method of finding a traveling companion. Organizations such as your local senior citizen center or historical society may also be able to help you.

Interests you especially enjoy, such as bridge or chess, may also provide leads. Call places where people participate in these kinds of activities, such as community centers, game stores, or clubs, and ask them to post your message.

Use bulletin boards to broaden possibilities. Put up your ad in the local market or drugstore, the library, the YWCA or YMCA, colleges or boarding schools, union halls, community or recreation centers, and public meeting places. Especially good places for notices are your local schools. Teachers often travel.

If you cannot go in person to put up your notice, call or send it by mail. Send your notice to the store manager, college president, head librarian or whoever else can either assist you or forward your letter to the appropriate person. Be creative! Someone, somewhere in your community would like to be your companion. If you find someone who is hesitant, consider that money may be the impediment to his or her joining you. Consider whether expenses could be shared. Traveling with someone you like is worth the extra money.

***How to Hire an Aide.*** If you have searched to no avail, don't give up. There are many places to hire someone to accompany you. Pick up your phone. Try your local high school, church or temple youth groups. Many teenagers are strong, responsible, and have a great zest for travel. Other places to contact include the local youth employment bureau, the student employment office or the dean of students of a college, your local home health offices or social services offices, visiting nurse associations, or hospitals—a nurse, nursing student or aide might like to join you.

*Cost of an Aide.* The cost of hiring a companion will vary. You may find someone willing to go for just his or her fare. Others may require room and board or even a salary. Don't be afraid to negotiate.

Be prepared with a list of questions when interviewing for a travel companion. You will want to know if the candidate is in good health and has the stamina for assisting you, has any experience in assisting a disabled person, and the disposition to deal with disabled people. Describe in detail the areas in which you will need help. Other pluses will be travel experience, knowledge of any foreign languages, assertiveness, and the ability to ignore other people staring or other difficult situations.

Many times a non-handicapped person may be afraid of you. No matter how good he or she may appear, he or she often has no experience in dealing with disabilities. Here are some questions to ask yourself:

Can I be by myself with this person or does he or she make me feel helpless?

Do I feel comfortable enough to ask for help and does he or she feel comfortable enough to have me refuse it?

Could I tell this person when he or she is treating me as handicapped rather than as a disabled person?

Can I talk to this person frankly about my needs, both emotional and physical?

Do we laugh together?

If you find someone who has the qualities you are looking for, you may also need to inform them of certain things. Don't take for granted that the person will know how to assist you. Tell him or her exactly where and when you will need assistance.

*Spend Time with Chosen Companion.* It is important that you spend time with your prospective companion. To see if you are compatible, go out to dinner, see a movie, or, if at all possible, take a day or weekend trip together. It is essential to learn each other's interests and frustration levels. This time together will give you the opportunity to explore whether you are truly right for one another. Compatibility is not just matching personalities, but a combining of lifestyles, idiosyncrasies and interests. Perhaps you are an early riser who has the most energy in the morning. It is important that you allot the morning for sightseeing so that you can rest in the afternoon. It would be a disaster for you to travel with someone who sleeps late and doesn't want to speak before ten o'clock. You will be spending a lot of time together and small annoyances can become intolerable. However, don't be so picky in choosing a traveling companion that you find yourself without one. The choice of a travel companion is not a lifetime commitment. Also, don't be too choosy about totally matching interests. A good companion is worth the compromise. Trade a museum for a shopping trip ... it's worth it. But don't go overboard on your compromises, because your time is more limited. While you are resting your companion can pursue personal interests. Any problems concerning lifestyles, idiosyncrasies and interests should be worked out before you go to avoid unpleasantness.

***I'm Going ... Maybe.*** Okay, you've decided you want to travel, but doubts and fears continue to plague you. This is natural since everyone should weigh such an important decision, especially first-time, disabled travelers. Your doubts are legitimate. Everything is harder for you. Conquering your doubts can be made more difficult by misinformed, overprotective and often biased opinions about what a disabled person can and cannot do. Just because your limbs don't work well doesn't mean your brain isn't functioning. A supportive person, who reinforces your status as an independent, thinking, free human being, is vital. Find one—it could make a difference between an expanding life and a static one.

The best way to deal with your anxieties, aside from having that essential, supportive friend, is to admit up front that there is a sound basis for some of them. For a better trip, acknowledge the fact that there are going to be problems and plan how to deal with them before you go.

Most of the problems you will encounter, besides the physical ones, often derive from sensitivity—too much by the disabled and too little by the public. You can't dictate the behavior of others, but you can control a situation by the way you react to it. For example, staring is a problem wherever you go; at home or abroad. People often stare at the disabled because they are curious, but their curiosity is not your problem. How you react to it is. Whether in Rome, Tokyo, or your own home town, you have every right to be there and someone's nosiness is immaterial. Remember, you're there to satisfy your own goals and priorities and no one else's. Besides, staring is not necessarily negative. Believe it or not, some of the starers are admiring you for your courage and tenacity. Assume this is true of all the people who stare at you and your discomfort becomes pride.

Embarrassment doesn't always emanate from others. Often we are our own worst enemies. Because we find some of our disabling conditions unsightly, we believe others do too. This internal stress makes it harder to dismiss and rationalize the reactions of others. We must deal with reality: some people cannot accept the unsightly side effects of disability such as drooling or twitching; frequently, the disabled are unable to accept these conditions themselves. It may not be ideal, but this is your life. If you are going to live with it, you must acknowledge the problem and deal with it. A thick skin and a will to survive are vital. It doesn't matter if you creep or shake; the point is to get there. Be practical; rather than missing the second floor of a museum, crawl up the stairs to see those inaccessible paintings!

Staring and discomfort are not confined to the disabled alone. The reaction that any traveler gets when he or she is visibly different from people he or she is visiting is influenced by superstitions and cultural idiosyncrasies. It's possible that you may encounter this cultural reaction. It could be because you are white, black, tall, short—as long as you are different. A black friend tells the story of how he was approached on the streets of Turkey by people who would wet their fingers and touch him to see if his color would rub off. If you should encounter such a reaction because of your disability, it may not be pleasant, but keep your sensitivity in check. It's not you as a person they are reacting to, but your disability. While rudeness is always intolerable, accept curiosity for what it is and don't take it as an insult.

On the other hand, don't assume that just because you are disabled in a foreign country you have to worry about whether you will be treated well. At the British Museum in London, employees are assigned to assist the touring disabled person, using special elevators so they won't miss anything. English people go out of their way to help; the guard at the Tower of London closed off the stairs to the crown jewels while a woman with a walker diligently made her descent. This kind of treatment is common in many countries including Denmark, Sweden, Norway and Italy, to name a few. The lure of the tourist dollar is teaching many other nations that the disabled must be accommodated.

Others' reactions to you are their problem. How you react is yours. For instance, some disabled people are grateful when help is offered while others are insulted that their independence is being questioned. Strangers have no way of knowing how you feel. Therefore, becoming angry and frustrated at their offer is unfair. It's enough to say, "No thank you."

My particular frustration occurs in restaurants. The waiter who ignores me and turns to ask my companion what I want doesn't really deserve courtesy. Although I would like to knock him over with my wheelchair, a dignified and carefully enunciated, "I would like ... " usually suffices. Although violence is tempting, it's bad for your digestion.

The various problems, personal and practical, that I have discussed so far are based on my own experience but are not meant to deter you. Knowing in advance the potential problems, and therefore, dealing with them, builds confidence. As a disabled person, I know that traveling for us takes more effort, both emotional and physical, but I also know that the rewards are worth the investment. Don't hesitate—GO!

# PLANNING YOUR TRIP

*I'm Going—But Where?* Now that you've decided to travel, the big question is where do you want to go? Has any special city or country captured your fancy? Will it be the countryside or metropolis? What about brushing up on a foreign language such as the French you took in high school? Whether it's sports, museums, shopping, food and wine, or historical sights, your trips should reflect your interests, not your disabilities. Your vacation can be centered on chess tournaments, photographing special events such as the New Year's Rose Bowl Parade, trying your luck at the casinos in Las Vegas, Monte Carlo, London or the Caribbean, or pursuing new additions to prized collections. Follow a whim: fly in hot air balloons. There's a ballooning trip in France through the beautiful Burgundian countryside that includes a stay in a late-seventeenth-century chateau. Let your imagination soar as you sort through a range of possibilities.

How much money you can afford for your trip is, of course, a key factor in decision making. Consider the total cost of different trips; divide the cost by the number of days you wish to spend on your trip to determine your daily expenditure. This estimate of daily expense will give you the opportunity to calculate the cost of side trips and extras, and find areas where trimming and tradeoffs can be made to allow you to do what you really want.

Traveling off-season can save you money. It's most expensive to travel to Europe from mid-June through mid-September and vice-versa for the Caribbean. You should be aware, however, that the "seasons" are considered desirable because the weather is at its best. On the other hand, at the height of the tourist season, you may have to contend with added crowds of your fellow travelers. A good time to visit is just before or after the "seasons." It will be cheaper and less congested. Make sure, though, that the natives aren't vacationing when you wish to visit. Many French people vacation in August, shutting down restaurants and shops and leaving a void in available services.

The amount of time you spend is not just a function of money. Other considerations include available vacation days and the special needs you may have. Will more than a week be too tiring? Do you have health care requirements that can't be arranged for away from home? What about missing physical therapy? These realities must be weighed carefully in determining where you will go, and for how long.

**Collecting Information.** Begin your planning by collecting information about the place or places that appeal to you. Forget for the moment that you have disabilities. Call or stop at your local travel agent to get brochures. Contact a library or bookstore and peruse the geography and travel sections. When looking, don't limit yourself to adult books. Books written for children often contain clearer descriptions and explanations. A trip that I took through the Amish country in Pennsylvania was greatly enhanced when our entire family prepared by reading an enlightening sixth grade book on the culture and sights. Other sources of background information are novels and histories.

If you don't have access to libraries or bookstores, write to the Forsythe Travel Library, P.O. Box 2975, Shawnee Mission, Kansas, 66201 for free catalogues and maps of places that interest you. Sometimes you can get ideas for your trip by watching television. The series "Elizabeth I," filmed in England, made me want to see Hampton Court, the scene of Elizabeth's childhood. When I visited this magnificent home, the sights I had seen while watching the series came to life. Scenes from the story kept coming to mind, bringing a sense of *déjà vu*.

For first-hand information, talk to friends and acquaintances about their trips. Everyone likes to share their travel memories. A friend who preceded me to London returned with facts on the accessibility of restaurants, hotels, stores, theaters, and historical attractions (see Publications from Federal Sources for Handicapped Travelers, p.*155*).

Once you have narrowed your search to a few places, contact the tourist bureaus of these countries. They usually offer travel brochures, maps and publicity on festivals, holidays, national discounts or rebates to promote tourism, and lists of hotels and other places to stay. For example, the Irish tourist agency will provide booklets on their famous "Bed n' Board" tours where you stay in farmhouses and private homes all over the country. See the appendix for listings of addresses of various foreign tourist bureaus to whom you can write as well as the Listing of Foreign Embassies and Consulates in the United States, p.*150*. To be sure that you will be sent exactly what you want and need, tell the agency when you wish to travel and what your disability is. They can then send you information pertinent to your trip.

The tourist agency may send you suggestions of other places to write for more information. The British Foreign Tourist Agency distributes copies of "British Information for the Disabled." This newspaper contains articles on people and organizations to contact for tours, cottage rentals, specially equipped cars, and other useful materials. When you write, include both the amount (if any) for the books and postage. If the charge is in foreign currency, call your bank and ask for the American equivalent.

Make your payment for charges and postage by personal check, bank check or money order to ensure a response. If you're not sure about the postage amount, ask your local post office.

Further listings for places to write are arranged alphabetically by country and city in the list of International Access Information, p.*129*.

***Traveling in the United States.*** Since the passage of federal legislation to aid the handicapped, and due to increased demands by the disabled, a greater effort to provide practical information, needed services, and improved accessibility is under way. Every state has a tourism department or bureau, Chamber of Commerce, and Easter Seal Foundation in its capital to assist you. All states and most major cities publish access guides outlining building standards and accommodations regarding things such as availability of elevators, location of bathrooms and widths of stalls, and policies on ramps and parking spaces. The Washington, D.C. access guide table of contents covers restaurants, museums, auditoriums, stadiums, banks, churches, government buildings, hotels and motels, libraries, department stores, galleries, recreational facilities, accessible sights of interest, theaters, movies and transportation. Not all books are so complete and some are outdated, but any information is useful to the disabled traveler. Addresses and sources of these guides are included in the appendix under Access Information in the United States, p *99*. If the city you are interested in is not in the listing, contact the state or local Chamber of Commerce.

A rule of thumb for choosing accessible places is, the more tourists who visit, the more likely there will be accommodations for the disabled. Large cities and warm spots such as Hawaii and Florida are used to dealing with all kinds of tourists and have made many provisions for the disabled. Disneyland and Disneyworld offer many attractions that can be viewed from a wheelchair. In addition to the availability of taxis, some large cities have made travel easier by providing special buses with hydraulic lifts that allow the wheelchair traveler to conveniently ride public transportation.

For those who enjoy the outdoors, steps are being taken to make parks, caverns, caves, forests, monuments, and battlefields accessible. Write to "Access National Parks," Superintendent of Documents, U.S. Government Printing Office, Washington, D.C. 20402 for information.

***Travel Terms.*** As you collect information for your trip, it is important to know travel industry terms to avoid misunderstandings. Some common terms you will encounter are:

*Modified American Plan*: Breakfast and dinner included.

*Continental Plan*: Breakfast of danish or croissant and coffee served.

*Breakfast Plan*: Full American-style breakfast served.

*Full Meal Plan*: All three meals are provided by the hotel.

*Dine Around Plan*: Dinners can be taken not only in the hotel in which you stay but also in other specified hotels.

*Meals in Flight*: Meals are served during flight by the airline. Since this is standard practice this is not a bonus. This may be an option, however, if you are traveling by an economy airline, which does not include food so that rates may be kept low.

*Courier*: The trip includes a guide who will travel with you throughout the trip or be available at the hotel to guide you and give you advice on your daily travels.

*Excursion Rates*: Special fares are available if the trip is made within a specified period of time, such as 21 to 30 days. There are no exceptions to the rules set down in this plan.

*Standby Travel*: Under this plan there are no reservations or seating. Whether you will depart on a particular flight will not be decided until shortly before takeoff when it is determined that a passenger with a reservation will not make the flight. While standby is cheaper, the obvious drawbacks of waiting make it undesirable for the disabled traveler. Airlines, under the regulations of the International Air Transport Association, may refuse to accept disabled passengers who have standby tickets.

*Transfers*: Transportation will be available to take you from the airport to your hotel and back.

*All Inclusive Land Portion*: The trip does not include air fares.

*Side Trips*: For an additional fee, a guided tour to sites not noted in the tour package will be provided. Although this may be convenient, it may be cheaper to wait until you arrive at your destination and hire a local guide.

*Charter Flights*: These are less expensive package tours arranged by travel agents and scheduled airlines that usually include a minimum air fare, hotel accommodations and optional meals. Many organizations offer charter trips to their members to specific places at selected times. Reputable organizations and travel agencies usually offer excellent values for the traveler. However, it is wise to check with your local consumer protection bureau to be sure. Also, to contain costs, airline seating is not deluxe and departure and arrival is scheduled for off-peak hours such as late at night.

**Climate.** A major consideration in deciding when and where to travel is the weather. If you suffer from arthritis or any ailment adversely affected by dampness, the rainy season anywhere is best avoided. Of course, no one can tell for sure what the weather will be like, but knowing the general weather patterns can prevent unpleasant surprises. Once you know what to expect, prepare for the unexpected. The sunshine the books promised can turn into showers. Plan agendas that can be substituted for outdoor activities. Or, be philosophical. A rainy day is great for resting up, writing home, keeping up with a journal, or mapping out future plans.

The section entitled Weather Conditions Around the World, p.*162*, includes temperature changes for each of the four seasons, temperature extremes, and the average monthly and annual precipitation rates. In addition, many large city newspapers list the average daily temperature in most cities around the world.

A final word about weather: be cautious but not too cautious. It is foolish to miss a chance to see something because the climate is not absolutely ideal. Not everywhere is like Hawaii. Even snow can be fun and beautiful if you know in advance and plan time, clothing and transportation accordingly.

**Places Not to Go.** China is one country that I would postpone visiting. Although it is trying to promote tourism, accommodations for the disabled are poor at this time. On the whole, facilities for the handicapped in China are about what they were in the United States in the 1940's.

A few joint venture hotels found in the largest cities (operated by the Chinese and a foreign country) may accommodate the disabled, but it is a tenuous situation. In Bejing, the Great Wall Hotel, Jing Guo Hotel, and the Bejing Toronto Hotel may have some accommodations for the disabled, but you must write to them and specifically inquire about what they offer. Facilities are quesitonable in Xi'an where the famous excavations draw many visitors. Travelers have found that hotels in small cities and the countryside are quite primitive and often have little or no housekeeping services.

Trains are a common way to travel in China. They have the hard seat section which you would want to avoid. Paying for the softer seats is well worth the money.

Thailand, a country much more modern than China, still has few services for the disabled. In many Far Eastern cultures, the family is responsible for all facets of life for the disabled and the government does nothing to provide services specifically for the disabled.

**Travel Agents.**  Even though you plan your own trip, you still need a travel agent to make certain arrangements for you. Aside from their knowledge of the mechanics of traveling, most of them are widely traveled themselves and can offer suggestions from personal experience. A good travel agent can assist you in getting where you want to go at the price you can afford, and, best of all, a travel agent doesn't cost you anything.

To find an agency that is reputable, you can ask friends for a recommendation, call your local Chamber of Commerce or Better Business Bureau, or look for a seal in the agency's window containing a globe with "ASTA" superimposed across it. This seal means that the travel agency belongs to the American Society of Travel Agents, which is located at 711 Fifth Avenue, New York, New York 10022. Another source of information regarding travel agents is the Society for the Advancement of Travel for the Handicapped (S.A.T.H.), 26 Court Street,

Brooklyn, New York 11242, a non-profit coalition of travel agents and tour operators who provide advice for the disabled traveler. (Travel agents who specialize in tours for the disabled are listed on p.157.)

I said before that a good travel agent can save you money. By this I mean more than just being able to arrange charters or book cheaper tours. In the United States, the Civil Aeronautics Board changes travel rates at will. Most travel agencies now have computers that allow them to obtain the latest and least expensive fares. What is the least expensive can sometimes be surprising. My agent cut my fare to Italy by advising me to fly to London and take the train the rest of the way. It cost less and I got to see scenery that I would have missed from the air. Besides coordinating your primary travel modes, your agent can also arrange car rentals and purchases for you.[1]

Read many guidebooks about the places you are going to visit. Fielding and Michelin are excellent guides but there are many other equally informative books on today's market. If you don't want to carry the books for ready reference, copy pertinent pages and take them along.

As you search for hotels, you will find greater opportunities in more modern hotels.[2] For example, forgo the quaint English boarding houses and opt for less traditional quarters that have fewer stairs. In more expensive hotels you will find bigger elevators, wider doorways, furniture that is easier to manipulate and on-site restaurants for when you are too tired to go out. Motels are preferable to hotels since they offer more space on the ground level. Since the travel industry is becoming more aware of the problems of the disabled, more new hotels and motels are meeting the needs of disabled travelers. Write to the major chains found in the yellow pages of your telephone directory and ask them which of their facilities is best for you. You can start by writing to Holiday Inn because one-third of the motels in that chain have adequate facilities, and Best Western Motels, which make an effort for wheelchair accessibility. Your

---

1. Different Ways to Travel, p.9. Hotel/Motel Chains with Accessible Units in the United States. Access Information in the United States.

2. International Access Books.

access guides will provide you with a listing of hotels and motels with special resources. However, be aware that since disabilities vary, hotels and motels claiming adequate facilities often do not meet everyone's needs.

When you or your travel agent make reservations at hotels, insist on a room near an elevator. If you are in a wheelchair or have trouble walking, proximity to the elevator will save you much energy. After a long day of sightseeing, this convenience will be greatly appreciated. Make sure your letter to the hotel mentions a need for this location.

You may want to try different travel experiences and use more than one transportation resource. You can mix planes, trains, cars or buses at your will. Just plan ahead. Your travel agent will be happy to make all reservations at no cost to you.

**Write for Access Information.** Although you read books, write to tourist bureaus, and see your travel agent, you still have one more step. Once you have decided where you will go, unless you have specific information on the hotels and sights you want to visit, it will be necessary to write for details regarding access.[3] When you write your letter, be brief, explain the facts and ask the necessary questions. Here is an example of such a letter and a list of questions you may select from:

Dear Sirs:

I am going to be in St. Louis from May 1 through 7. I am looking forward to staying in a hotel that will accommodate me and my wheelchair. Could you please answer the following questions for me:

Is the entrance to the hotel flat or is there a ramp for access

Is the lobby level, or must you go up stairs to reach an elevator

Is the elevator large enough for a wheelchair

If the elevators are self-service, can you reach the buttons from a wheelchair

Are the numbers on the elevator in braille or do you have a bell signal for floors

---

3. Access information in the United States. International Access Books.

Are the restaurants, coffee shop, and bar wheelchair
  accessible
Is room service available
Is there a garage or valet parking
Is there a space reserved for handicapped parking
Are the doorways in the room at least 32 inches wide
Are sinks and vanities 27 inches or lower
Are there telephones in the room
Are the telephones equipped with braille code, raised
  block letters and volume control
Do rooms have a bolt-lock on the door
Is there a chain that can be reached from my wheelchair
May furniture be easily moved for mobility with a
  wheelchair in the room
What are the heights of the dresser drawers
Are the closet hangers low
Are there grab bars around the toilet and shower
Is the toilet raised
Do they have "roll-in showers" so wheelchairs can easily
  enter or are there seats within the bathtub
Are there light and TV controls near the bed
Are there soda and ice machines on the same floor
Is it possible to have a room located near the elevator

**Passports.** Since getting a passport can be a time consuming
process, it should be one of the first priorities on your list of
things to do (see Visas and Passports, p.*160*). Your passport is an
important document. It is your legal identification abroad that
proves you are an American citizen. Therefore, never lend it to
anyone and protect it from spills, being written on or muti-
lated. Most countries require a passport however, it is not illegal
to travel without a passport in the Panama Canal Zone, Puerto
Rico, Guam, American Samoa, Virgin Islands, Canada, Bermuda
or the Caribbean countries. Although you don't need a passport, you are required to have a tourist card to travel to Belize
(British Honduras), the British West Indies, Costa Rica, the
Dominican Republic, El Salvador, the French West Indies,
Guatemala, Haiti, Jamaica, Mexico, Nicaragua and Panama.
Regardless, it is still prudent to carry a passport since it is the
best proof you have of your American citizenship, and you
never know under what circumstances you will need it.

If you have a passport, check the date it was issued, since it is only valid for ten years. If your passport expires near the date you are going to travel, get a new one before you go. Although they can be renewed abroad, it is complicated, time consuming and may delay your journey.

To obtain a passport, you must have a head and shoulder photograph taken that is no larger than three inches square with a matte finish. You cannot take the picture yourself or in a photo booth. Check the yellow pages of a telephone directory for a list of photographers who specialize in passport photos. Smile when you get your picture taken, as it's the image you portray to all foreign officials. You will also need proof of citizenship, which can be a birth certificate, affidavit of birth, an old passport or a baptismal certificate. If born in another country, your naturalization papers are necessary. You can obtain your passport through U.S. Passport offices in New York, Boston, Philadelphia, Washington, D.C., Los Angeles, San Francisco, Seattle, Chicago, Miami, New Orleans, Honolulu, Detroit, Houston, and Stamford, Connecticut. You may also apply for a passport from the clerk of any federal court, authorized state court, and many post offices throughout the nation. Applications may also be obtained from travel agents or international airline offices. You must appear in person for your first passport. It will cost you $35 plus $7 handling fee for a passport issued for ten years. To renew a passport, you may write to any of the U.S. Passport offices or the Passport Office, Washington, D.C. 20524 and be sure to enclose the $42 to cover costs, your old passport, and two recent, identical photographs which you have signed. In 1993 these prices will no longer be in effect.

When you write for a passport, it will only be issued in the name of the old passport. If you have married and wish to change the name on your passport, you must send a copy of your marriage certificate or a copy of the name-change court document.

It is possible to obtain a single passport under the husband's name for an entire family. This is not advisable because the husband may have to return home for business or other reasons. Also, if the family wants to see two different events in one day, it is not possible because half the family would not have proof of identification which can be requested at any time. Spend the additional money and have the wife take out a passport in her own name.

Passports are essential to smooth traveling. You must keep your passport with you at all times. Many countries require hotels to keep a record of where their guests come from and will ask you to leave your passport at the desk at night and pick it up in the morning. Beware of theft. Thousands of passports are stolen each year becuase they are very valuable on the black market. If your passport is stolen or lost, follow instructions on how to rectify the situation (see If Disaster Strikes, p.86).

Passport pouches, which hang around your neck, may be purchased in some luggage stores. However, to protect my passport, I made a small case to hold it which I can wear pinned under my clothes. To make this bag you need not be a seamstress or a tailor. Here are the directions: Buy a strong material and velcro tape that sticks together. To make a 3" by 6" bag, cut material 5" by 16" long. Fold material and sew sides one inch from the edge at the top, fold over each open edge an inch twice so the cut edges are hidden. Sew across each side. Turn bag right-side out. Sew velcro, making sure tape is sewn correctly to either side of the inside of the top, so when pushed together, the tape sticks and the bag stays closed.

**Visas.** A visa is a stamp that most countries put on your passport, but a few countries put on a piece of paper. About sixty percent of countries require a visa to allow you to cross their borders (see Visas and Passports, p.160). Visas are not necessary for travel to the Caribbean Islands, Latin America, and Western Europe, but are essential in most other areas of the world. Your travel agent will be glad to ascertain whether you will need a visa. You must obtain your visa before you leave the United States by applying in person or by mail from a foreign embassy in the United States (see Foreign Embassies and Consulates in the United States, p.150).

**Customs.** Your declaration of goods when passing through

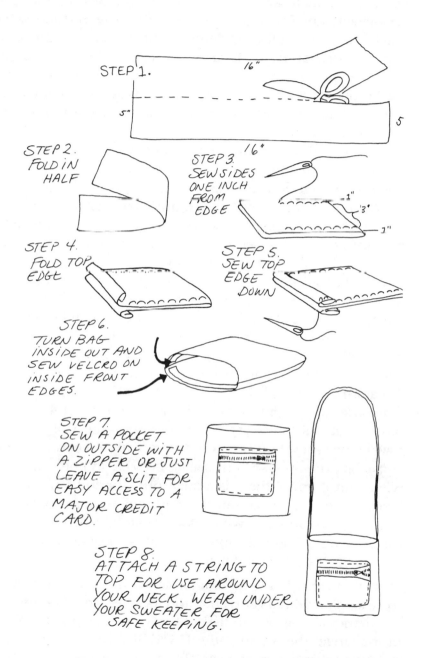

STEP 1.   16"

5"                                          5

STEP 2.
FOLD IN
HALF

STEP 3.   16"
SEW SIDES
ONE INCH
FROM
EDGE
1"
3"
1"

STEP 4.
FOLD TOP
EDGE

STEP 5.
SEW TOP
EDGE
DOWN

STEP 6.
TURN BAG
INSIDE OUT AND
SEW VELCRO ON
INSIDE FRONT
EDGES.

STEP 7.
SEW A POCKET
ON OUTSIDE WITH
A ZIPPER OR JUST
LEAVE A SLIT FOR
EASY ACCESS TO A
MAJOR CREDIT
CARD.

STEP 8.
ATTACH A STRING TO
TOP FOR USE AROUND
YOUR NECK. WEAR UNDER
YOUR SWEATER FOR
SAFE KEEPING.

customs is usually accepted at face value. However, if the agent spot-checks and find that you have under-declared goods, you will be subject to a fine. In some countries, such as the Soviet Union, undeclared goods are confiscated. If the violation is large enough, you could be arrested, detained and subject to legal proceedings. It is wise to declare everything that you are bringing into a country. If items are unclaimed and then discovered, you risk arrest.

Some countries prohibit or restrict certain goods.[4] Many countries will not let you bring in weapons or firearms, which might also include fireworks and knives; others require permits at time of entrance. Some countries don't allow alcohol to be brought in. Check before you go with your travel agent or the countries' embassies (see Foreign Embassies and Consulates in the United States, p.150). Certain countries ban goods from other countries (for example, Libya will not allow goods to be imported from Israel or other countries that trade with Israel). Literature is sometimes banned for political, religious or moral reasons. China bans anti-China literature. Russia restricts the importation of religious articles, such as bibles, and many countries refuse to allow the importation of pornographic literature.

In order to prevent disease, all countries restrict the importation of plants, foods, vegetables and meats, and all countries have some restrictions on pets. Check with the country's consulate before you take your seeing-eye dog to find out if they will admit it and if there is a quarantine period. An excellent brochure listing all countries' requirements and policies is *Traveling With Your Pet*, which is available from Animalport, Air Cargo Center, Kennedy International Airport, Jamaica, New York 11430. It costs one dollar.

*Money.* If you plan to go to a foreign country it is imperative to be familiar with its currency and its worth in comparison to U.S. money (see appendix list entitled Currency, p.158). The rate of exchange, the amount the U.S. dollar will buy in foreign currency, changes every day. These rates are posted at hotel

---

4. *Super Traveler*, Saul Millery, Holt, Rhinehart and Winston, New York.

desks, in banks, and often near cashiers in restaurants. It is important for shopping, eating in restaurants, and paying hotel bills to understand the currency of the different countries you will be visiting. The best way to become familiar with a particular foreign currency is to order a $20 trip pack in that currency from your local bank. This pack will include a combination of currency, bills and coins, and a chart giving approximate conversion rates. This pack allows you to practice using the actual coins and currency so you can be quite adept at it before you leave. This familiarity with foreign money makes it less likely you will be cheated on prices or change, and you will be less apt to fumble and drop coins or bills that are difficult to pick up. Since they take approximately four weeks to arrive, order trip packs as soon as you know where you will be traveling. Another aid for converting currency is Fielding's "World Currency Converter," a sliding scale that aligns U.S. currency with foreign currency, and that can be found in many bookstores.

***How to Take Your Money.*** Most of your money should be converted into travelers checks (American Express, Bank America). Make two copies of the serial numbers of your travelers checks. Keep one list with a friend at home who can be reached easily in an emergency. Pack your original list and a copy in two different places, so if your checks are lost or stolen you have a better chance of locating the serial numbers for replacement purposes. In the section entitled If Disaster Strikes, p. 86, there are suggestions about what to do if your travelers checks are lost or stolen. Do not carry your travelers checks or money all in one place. Prudent travelers pin their cash inside their clothes or wear money belts. Others lock their extra checks and money in their suitcases. The safest method is to leave the majority of your money and travelers checks in the hotel safe.

Cash travelers checks in a bank rather than at the hotel, which may charge expensive conversion fees. You may also want to carry personal checks as security to know that you have additional money. A section on "What to Do When You

Run Out of Money" is found on p.*94*.

It's necessary for disabled travelers to carry extra money because traveling as a disabled person is more expensive than for the average traveler. Take at least $100 per day. When I arrived in Denmark, I discovered people in wheelchairs could not use public transportation. My only alternatives were to take taxis everywhere, rent a car, or rent a car with a chauffeur. All these choices were unexpected expenses. I usually carry $20 in one dollar bills so I have money ready for tipping (see When You Get There, p.*72*).

Other additional expenses may occur if you are tired after a day of sightseeing and are too exhausted to go out to dinner. Eating in the hotel or calling room service will be more expensive but certainly worth the convenience.

If you are in a wheelchair, tipping is more costly for you than the average traveler because you need more assistance. This includes help with your luggage at train stations and airports, getting a taxi driver to lift your wheelchair in and out of the car, lifting you if you need assistance, calling a reputable taxi firm and often negotiating rates with taxi drivers. People deserve generous trips for the indispensable help.

In taxis, two bags usually go free, and your wheelchair will be counted as one of those bags. They will charge extra if you have more than one bag. The more aware and sophisticated you appear, the less likely you will be taken advantage of by others. Often management at restaurants and hotels have arrangements with taxi cab companies. If these firms don't turn out to be reputable, they don't call them again.

You may have to pay additional costs for your wheelchair. Before you leave home, whenever possible, you should check with your travel agent or the airline, train, bus and limousine services for the cost of transporting your wheelchair. Usually in foreign countries taxi rates are an unknown commodity. Before you enter the taxi, find out how much the driver charges for your wheelchair as well as for the ride. Often the maitre d' in a restaurant, someone from your hotel, or an employee from the site you are visiting will negotiate the terms for you. Sometimes you will be charged for your wheelchair as if it were an extra person.

**Clothes.**  Although deciding what clothes to take seems befuddling, don't despair. Make a list of all the clothes you think you will need for your activities in a particular climate. Go over the list and eliminate clothes you really don't need or that will wrinkle so badly that they are better off left at home. Wash and wear clothes and knits are ideal for traveling because they require minimal care and they wrinkle the least. After paring down your list, see what you need to buy to complete your wardrobe. Since the average sightseer is not traveling as part of a fashion show, it is not necessary to spend much money on clothes. As long as you look neat and clean and are comfortable, you are "clothes-ready" for traveling.

Pick a color scheme and choose your clothes accordingly so that you can mix and match outfits for variety. This approach works equally well for women and men. Dark, simple clothes are excellent in colder climates and in large cities as they are suitable for more occasions and show less soil. However, in tropical climates, take white, bright, light clothes.

What to wear in large cities is sometimes perplexing for women. If you are most comfortable sightseeing in a pantsuit or dressier slacks, you will be appropriately dressed in any city. Skirts and blouses or a simple dress with a jacket are also suitable. Those who suffer from ailments that are influenced by damp weather should dress warmly. Bathing suits and shorts are frowned upon in cities regardless of how warm the weather.

A woman will have adequate clothing if she takes one suit (skirt or pants), one skirt, two blouses and a dress. Add to this list a pair of slacks and sweater and you have your basic wardrobe. Don't forget six pairs of pantyhose, three sets of underwear (bras, panties, slips), nightgowns and a robe. You may want to use a raincoat as a robe to save room in your suitcase. Take a pocketbook for day use and a dress bag for the evening. Your everyday bag should have a zipper compartment for ease in finding items and to guard against loss. Try and take clothes for daytime wear that can be dressed up in the evening with a scarf or a simple piece of jewelry. Take two comfortable pairs of shoes; fit not fashion is important. Add a pair of dress shoes for evening wear. Take a trenchcoat with a lining if the weather warrants a coat. You may find a fold-up, plastic raincoat useful in warmer climates where a coat is unnecessary.

A man can easily travel with one suit, two pairs of slacks and a sport jacket. If your suit is a solid color the jacket can be worn with a pair of slacks from a different outfit. Pack six shirts unless you intend to take drip-dry shirts and then three will be adequate. Add to your list: six pairs of socks, three sets of underwear, one pair of pajamas, a robe, some handkerchiefs, five ties, a sweater and two comfortable pairs of shoes. A raincoat can be used for more than one purpose.

Never take an item of sentimental value, regardless of how inexpensive it is, if it can't be replaced. If you must take expensive jewelry and do not plan to wear it at all times, do not leave it lying around your hotel room where it can be accidentally swept away during cleaning or become a temptation for theft. Put it in the hotel safe. Expensive jewelry also makes you a target for robbery on the streets and is best left at home.

**Traveling In Two Different Climates.** If you plan to travel in two different climates where you will need two sets of clothes, simply make two lists. Pack the clothes you will be wearing first. Mail your second wardrobe to a hotel where you will be staying with your name and date of arrival clearly marked on the outside of the packages. Mark "hold for arrival" in a conspicuous area. After you are finished with the first set of clothes, mail them home.

**Luggage.** Soft luggage is best for several reasons. Most important, it is the easiest to lift and you may have to carry it yourself. Also, soft luggage holds about half again as much as hard luggage. It should be packed to slightly bulging so clothes stay tightly packed and are less prone to wrinkling. The disadvantage of soft luggage is that it is more likely to tear and show abuse.

Don't take more than one piece of luggage which can fit across the top of your wheelchair comfortably. Take a carry-on bag to hold your drugs, cosmetics and a change of clothes. By traveling lightly, you will not be encumbered by having to transport a lot of luggage.

Put baggage labels with your name and address on all your suitcases. Attach a business card or a note with your home address inside your luggage in case your outside tags are ripped off. It is also prudent to place a piece of paper with your next destination on top of your clothes in case your luggage is lost. Airline personnel will then know where to forward your luggage. If you affix your initials in adhesive or colored tape on the outside of your luggage, it will be easier to identify on the luggage racks, lessening the chances for a mix-up with someone else's similar luggage.

Cloth bags that attach to your wheelchair are useful. Make a bag similar to your passport bag, but add ties so you can attach it to the arms of your wheelchair. I have found that one bag, 15" x 16" finished size, is sufficient to hold items that I want to use every day. It shouldn't be used to hold a passport, travelers checks or large amounts of money. It will hold makeup, snacks, change for tips, kleenex, tobacco, maps or travel guides, or anything else you would like to reach easily. A similar bag, about 18" x 18" finished size, could be tied to the handles of the back of your wheelchair to store purchases or more cumbersome items that you want to carry. If someone else is pushing you, it could be an ideal place to store your camera. When making these bags, follow the directions given on page 27 for passport bags. Cut the material two inches wider than the finished size on the sides so that you have a one-inch seam; allow four extra inches on the top where you will attach the tape to close the bag.

***Airline Luggage Restrictions.*** In traveling within the United States, luggage is now restricted by size, not weight. A passenger may check two free pieces of luggage plus a carry-on bag. When traveling abroad, each airline has a different policy about luggage and the cost of taking your wheelchair. Many airlines will carry your wheelchair for free. Check the chart, "Services Provided for Disabled Passengers," on page 56 to see if

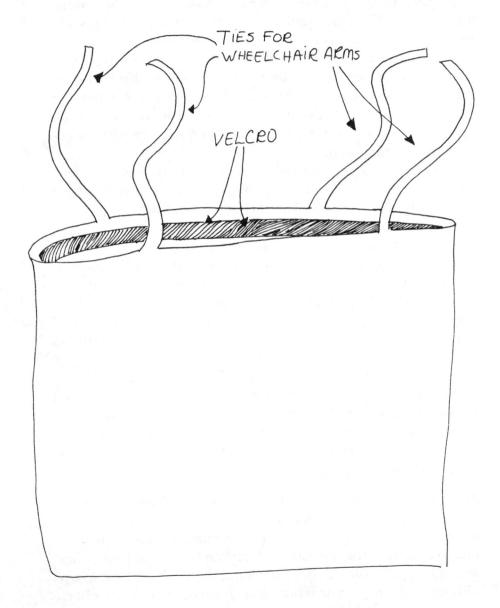

TIES FOR
WHEELCHAIR ARMS

VELCRO

there is a fee. A rule of thumb is that you are only entitled to two pieces of luggage, 62" height plus width plus length, which are commonly called "two suiters," or 62 pounds per bag. In addition, your carry-on bag must fit under your seat.

***Additional Items to Take.*** Include in your packing items you find relaxing. If you like to play Backgammon or Scrabble take along the small versions of these games designed for travelers. If you enjoy needlepoint, take a needlepoint project for long plane or train rides or for something to do if you are forced to remain in your room. If you enjoy reading, pack a few books. Make sure you include a flashlight since, in many countries, reading lights are poor or inconveniently placed.

There are some other helpful items to take long. A language dictionary will be useful in country where the people don't speak your language. Try to learn some useful phrases before you leave home (see Tourist Vocabulary Tips, p. *164*). People will appreciate your effort to use their language even if you mispronounce the words. Learning the names of some foods is especially helpful because you can read a menu and point to what you want even if you are embarrassed to speak a different language.

For those who have difficulty with foreign languages, make foreign phrase vocabulary cards on small index cards. Type or print the phrase in English on one side and in the foreign language on the other side. Carry blank cards and have an English speaking person write other necessary phrases for you when you get to a foreign country.

You will need an adapter for your American appliances in most European countries because they use 220 volts and we use 110. The latest hair dryers and electric razors have adapters built in and you may want to invest in one. It may be more convenient for your trip to switch from an electric razor to a standard razor or a cordless, battery operated one. However, most deluxe hotels have 110 volt outlets, the same as in the United States.

Pack a bar of soap, which many hotels outside the United States do not provide. Many Americans take toilet paper, since in many other countries it is rough and very unlike what you are accustomed to at home.

You may also find a travel alarm clock helpful in getting up early to make the most of each day and to ensure that you make travel connections. Wake-up calls by hotels can be unreliable.

If you smoke, pack your maximum limit of cigarettes, cigars or pipe tobacco because tobacco products are much more expensive outside the United States. Also, it may be difficult to locate your brand.

A must in packing is an immersion heater coil (and an unbreakable cup), an inexpensive and wonderful gadget for heating water. You will appreciate it when you want to make coffee as soon as you wake up, for making broth to arrest your hunger between meals, or hot cocoa to relax you enough to sleep. You will need an adapter for this appliance, too.

Scotch tape can be a lifesaver. It can be used for the many functions it serves at home and also for a quick clothing repair such as fixing a hem. Don't forget a small sewing kit or, at least, spools of black and white thread and a needle.

Be prepared to repair your wheelchair, walker, cane or crutches. If a tool kit came with your wheelchair, take it along. If you don't have tools, try to buy a set from a store that handles your brand of wheelchair, or write to the manufacturer. If all else fails, make your own tool kit. You can make most wheelchair repairs with a wrench, pliers, and a Phillips screwdriver. If you can't make the repairs yourself, you can usually find someone willing to lend you a hand, or you can contact a local garage and ask for a mechanic to assist you.

If you use a cane, crutches or a walker, pick up a replacement set of rubber caps that fit on the bottom to replace the old ones when they become worn or lost.

Make yourself a small laundry kit and include packets of Woolite, a small clothesline to use in bathrooms, and some small, plastic clothespins. You may wish to use a hotel's laundry service, and, if you are in a big city, there are usually laundries and dry cleaners nearby. However, it is more convenient and time-saving, and less costly, to launder your clothes yourself.

***How to Pack.*** Packing can be a simple process if you make lists of the clothes and the extra things you are taking. A week before you leave check to see if anything needs to go to the cleaners or is in need of repair. Launder the clothes you will pack and try to wear outfits that you are not taking. I find it useful to pack alone so I can concentrate without being interrupted. Take your list and lay all your clothes out on the bed. Plan to wear your heaviest clothes when traveling, so put them in a separate area. I prefer to pack with tissue paper to avoid wrinkling. Lay a blouse, dress or shirt flat and place a piece of tissue paper on top; then fold as you normally would and you will find that clothes arrive neater. The best way to get wrinkles out of woolen clothes on the road is to hang them in the bathroom when you take a steamy shower or bath.

While packing, try to keep clothes level and secure. If you are packing suits, place the first folded area to the right. In the next layer, put the folded area to the left so that the clothes remain at an even height. Place the heaviest clothes, such as shoes, on the bottom. Fold underwear in half and roll it up so it can be used to fill empty spaces. The tighter you pack clothes the more winkle free they will remain. When you are completely finished, lock your suitcase. If your lock is broken or your suitcase is old, tie a baggage strap or heavy rope around your suitcase. This isn't tacky, it's smart. In fact, the owner of the store where I bought my luggage told me he always ties his luggage to discourage theft. Last, weigh your bag. Try and stay five pounds under the maximum to allow for items you may buy abroad and carry home.

***Cosmetics.*** Make a list of the items you wish to bring just as you did with clothes. Eliminate anything you are uncertain about since you will tend to pack too much. Besides, you can buy cosmetics anywhere. Take small quantities to waste as little space as possible. Transfer your cosmetics or liquids into plastic containers if they come in glass. Never pack liquids with your clothes, in case containers leak. Pack them in a plastic bag or cosmetics case.

***Diets.*** Don't allow special diets to interfere with your trip. You can take care of yourself and still have a good time. If you need to adhere to a special diet during flight, see the airplane section in Different Ways to Travel, p. 53 , which will tell you what is available and how to make arrangements. You can stick to your diet while traveling with a little ingenuity and great restraint. If you have an allergy to certain foods or need a salt-free diet, inform the waiter. If you don't speak the language, before you leave home, obtain a language book for the country or countries you are going to visit and make cards that you can present at meals telling of your food allergies or diet restraints. If you can speak the language you might call restaurants ahead of time and ask if they can accommodate you.

If you must diet to maintain your weight, here are some suggestions. Lose some weight before you leave so you can eat more while traveling. If you are determined to control your weight, every country has food you can eat without feeling guilty. Try and eat before you go sightseeing for additional strength and because the exercise will burn off more calories. Drink wine instead of beer. Eat less spicy foods since spices make you thirstier and you will retain more fluids. If courses are as large as they are in Germany and Austria, just order the main dish. Beware of very strong coffee; you may find yourself adding large amounts of sugar. Pass up fancy pastries and cakes and adopt the European habit of eating cheese and fruit at the end of a meal. Or better yet, skip dessert and sip the many delicious teas and coffees that foreign restaurants have to offer.

Order broiled fish or chicken whenever possible, without breading or sauces. You will still be exposed to some wonderful cuisine. Order fresh salads without dressing and bring your own individually packaged diet salad dressing, sold in most markets in the United States. In France, look for restaurants that feature "nouvelle cuisine," the popular new method of French cooking that emphasizes steamed vegetables, veal, chicken and fish, with herb dressings rather than the traditional French sauces. Portions are small in France and England, which should help with your diet. If traveling in France, you will note that the natives often have yogurt for dessert, since they believe it cleans the palate. Tourists prefer the heavy French pastries. Go native.

The following Weight Watchers Magazine "Five Mini-Dictionaries for Dieters Abroad" should be helpful:

## FIVE MINI-DICTIONARIES FOR DIETERS ABROAD

| English | French | German | Italian | Spanish |
|---|---|---|---|---|
| broiled | rôti | gegrillt | ala griglia | a la parrilla |
| steamed | cuit à la vapeur | gedünstet | bolliti | al vapor |
| without butter | sans bourre | ohne Butter | senza burro | sin mantequilla |
| without sugar | sans sucre | ohne Zucker | senza zucchero | sin azúcar |
| without salt | sans sel | ohne Salz | senza salato | sin sal |
| margarine | margarine | Margarine | margarina | margarina |
| saccharine | saccharine | Saccharin | saccarina | sacarina |
| sauce on the side, please | la sauce à part, s'il vous plaît | ohne Sauce, bitte (without sauce); nur ein Löffel Sauce (only one spoonful of sauce*) | sugo de parte, per favore | la salsa aparte, por favor |
| rare, medium, well-done | saignant, à point, bien cuit | halbroh, halb-gebraten, durch-gebraten | al sangue, cottura media, ben cotto | poco cocinado, media cocinado, bien cocinado |
| skim milk | du lait écrémé | fettarme Milch | latte scremato | leche descrema |
| mineral water | de l'eau minérale | Mineral-wasser | acqua minerale | agua mineral |
| dry, white wine | du vin blanc sec | herber Wein | vino bianco secco | vino blanco seco |
| juice | du jus | der Saft | succo | el jugo |
| low-calorie meal | un repas à basse calorie | Schlankheitskost | un pranzo con poche caloria | una comida de pocas calorías |
| low calorie specialty | une spécialité à basse calorie | Schlankheitsmenu | | una especialidad de pocas calorías |
| I'm on a diet | Je suis au régime | Ich mache sin Schlankheitskur | Io sono a dieta | Estoy a dieta |

* For some reason a request for sauce or gravy served separately causes great confusion in most German restaurants. It's better to request a meal without sauce or with one (ein) or two (zwei) spoonfuls. Weight Watchers Magazine, July 1982, p. 16, Reprinted with permission.

***Take Some Food With You.*** It is important to pack items that add to your comfort. Since medication and your physical condition may require you to eat at unconventional times in the country you are visiting, it is important to take some food along. These snacks may also become small meals when you don't feel well and have no desire to leave your bed. Pack a small jar of peanut butter, crackers, teabags or coffee bags, or packages of cocoa if caffeine is off limits. Include a package of hard candy to take away the aftertaste of unpleasant medications. If you are uncomfortable going to a bar or café alone, take a corkscrew so you can enjoy wine in your room.

***Planning for Bargain Shopping.*** If you plan to shop for bargains on your trip, it helps to be prepared. Do some research, so no one can take advantage of you. Find out what products the places you are going to visit are famous for: Appalachian quilts, Hawaiian coral and pearls, Swiss watches and clocks, Chinese ivory and jade, or Danish sweaters. Check the prices on these items in catalogs, department stores, and specialty stores before you leave home. Then, for instance, when you shop for a sweater in Denmark, you will know how much a similar sweater would cost in the United States and whether you're getting a bargain.

Even if you aren't interested in buying something for yourself, you may want to offer to shop for a close friend or relative. A friend of mine was thrilled when I was able to add to her collection of Royal Danish Christmas plates for $20, when the same plate would have cost her $57 at home. Of course, to avoid problems make it clear that shipping is at their risk and not yours, if goods are broken or stolen.

If you plan to bring home liquor or wine specialties from a foreign country, buy small bottles at home and sample them to see what you like. Then, instead of standing bewildered in a liquor store or duty free market, you will be able to make your purchases wisely.

***Mail.*** Sending mail to and from abroad can be made easier and more reliable by planning ahead. While at home, type or write labels for the postcards and letters you want to send. The advantage is that you can write at your leisure and will have needed information, such as zip codes, at your disposal, and will be less apt to leave someone off your list.

Before you leave home, write the names of hotels, addresses and the dates you will be staying for friends and relatives who may be writing to you. To make sure you receive your mail, check the post office at home for an estimate of how long delivery will take and note it on the paper with the addresses.

If you are a member of American Express, you may receive mail at their offices throughout the world. Contact an American Express office for addresses.

Remind your friends to print, making addresses easier to read and ensuring that you receive their letters. Also, have them print "hold for arrival" or "please forward," whichever is appropriate to the schedule of where you may be at the time.

You will need the correct amount of postage for mailing cards and letters back home. The concierge at your hotel will stamp and mail letters and cards for you with the correct postage. If there is no concierge, ask at the hotel desk if there is someone who will help you with your mailing. Hotel lobbies usually have mailboxes.

**Insurance.** There are many insurance options available for travelers. First, check your homeowner's policy or apartment renter's insurance to see if your luggage, camera and other valuables are covered if lost or stolen away from home. Check your medical insurance and see if it provides ample coverage. If your property or medical insurance is inadequate, explore options. Over-the-counter policies are sold at airports to insure you if your plane crashes. Comprehensive travel insurance, sold either as a package or with some options, is available through your travel agent or ARM Coverage, Inc. (9 East 37th Street, New York, New York 10016, 212-683-2622). Among the different types of travel insurance coverage available are: trip cancellation by airlines or tour operators; expenses incurred as a result of hijacking or an airline employee strike; reimbursement for emergency expenses if your luggage is misdirected or delayed (although airlines often pay these expenses); evacuation assistance if doctors determine you must be transported elsewhere for emergency medical treatment; and trip cancellation insurance because of illness or death of yourself, family or an unrelated companion traveling with you.

A typical comprehensive package might cost about $75 per person for a ten-day trip and provide $47,000 worth of coverage, divided into amounts for the coverage options previously mentioned.

Read carefully the section of any insurance policy application marked "exclusions." It will often state that you will not be covered for a pre-existing illness if you must return home, which gets you into a gray area. Insurance companies will usually cover an illness you had previously if medical records show that the condition has not changed and your medication had not been changed on your last visit to the doctor. However, you must have a doctor who treats you abroad write that it is upon his or her advice that you must return home. Airline and hotel penalties for cancellations can be very expensive, so you may want to check with your travel agent about trip cancellation insurance. It will cost you about $4 for every $100 of coverage. Only buy as much coverage as you need to fly home and to pay for additional expenses that would be incurred from cancellation.

Being more knowledgeable makes for a more successful trip. Take a notebook or travel journal (that can be purchased at most stationery stores) and jot down information that you will want to use when you travel. This journal can be part of your travel diary if you decide to write about your travel experiences.

# STAYING HEALTHY WHILE TRAVELING

## by Dr. Margaret Hayes

When you first plan your trip make sure to visit your doctor. Discuss your plans and any problems that might arise because of your condition. Make sure that the temperature and altitude of your destination won't cause any particular health problems.

The U.S. Public Health Service and some foreign countries insist that you be immunized against certain diseases. Ask your doctor about preventative measures, such as tetanus innoculations, that might be useful. Have your injections in advance to avoid a negative reaction that might be detrimental to your trip.

Small problems can make your trip unpleasant. Take care of ingrown toenails, corns and dental cavities before you leave. Think over your past year's health experiences. Have you had to consult your doctor for any problems that might recur? Often urinary tract infections, vaginal infections, migraine headaches, hemorrhoids, excessively heavy or painful menstrual periods, or fluid retention can reappear and disturb your trip. Ask advice for allergies, diarrhea and motion sickness. Your doctor can give you a prescription to take if a problem arises.

Have your doctor write a report stating your exact problems and limitations. This report should include copies of your current prescriptions including generic names and doses. Add your doctor's and dentist's addresses and telephone numbers to your medical write-up in case it is necessary to contact them. Carry two copies of your medical documents: one with your passport and one in your suitcase.

***Some General Hints while Traveling.*** Your medication requires as much care as you do. Keep your medication in its original container that must be well labeled in case you have to reorder. Pills are easiest to carry since liquids can spill and capsules can be damaged by weather extremes. Carry liquids in small, plastic bags. Always carry your medicines in your carry-on luggage in case your suitcase gets lost or delayed. Take enough medicine to last a few more days than your trip in case unavoidable delays change your plans.

Try and get enough rest while you are traveling. A lack of sleep, jet lag and strange foods can make anyone susceptible to illness. A frequent transcontinental traveler gave me some good advice. Take a nap as soon as you arrive at your hotel. It does wonders for jet lag and the general tired feeling that occurs while traveling long distances.

***What to Pack.*** Besides taking prescription medicines, it is wise to include the following:

Small tissue packs.

Towelettes—they will not only refresh you when you are sightseeing but hand cleanliness also prevents many illnesses.

Soap—you will be amazed at what passes for this product in other countries.

Toilet paper—a neat trick is to have half used rolls of toilet paper which can be flattened for packing and easily stored in a pocketbook or suitcase.

For pain—aspirin, buffered tablets or a non-aspirin compound will be helpful.

For indigestion—antacid tablets are helpful.

For diarrhea—antidiarrhetic medicine is a necessity.

For constipation—carry laxative tablets or packages.

For allergies—a nasal spray or antihistamine is a good precaution.

For motion sickness—buy over-the-counter medications or prescriptions for adhesive patches that go on the skin behind your ears.

For infections—if you are susceptible, your doctor may prescribe a broad spectrum of antibiotics.

For skin care—powder, petroleum jelly, lotion or cream containing hydro-cortisone is useful for sunburn and other rashes. Many forget that while you are sightseeing you often spend much time in the sun.

For insect bites—repellents are essential, especially in the tropics.

For footcare—antifungal powder is useful for those who have problems with their feet.

For eyecare—if your glasses are essential, take an extra pair. Don't forget a copy of your prescription, sunglasses and a small bottle of soothing eyedrops. If you wear contact lenses, don't forget your cleansing and soaking solution.

For first aid—bandaids, small gauze dressings, first aid cream, adhesive tape and corn plasters are wise to have along. An ace bandage is good for a sore or sprained wrist or ankle and can also be used to hold a broken suitcase together.

For ear care—those who wear a hearing aid should carry extra batteries.

Menstrual supplies—even if your period is not due during your trip, take supplies as well as medication for dysmenorrhea if necessary.

For contraception—birth control pills, diaphragm, prophylactics, foam or cream must be taken; they may not be available in other countries.

For insomnia—bring sleeping pills if you have trouble sleeping in strange beds.

Thermometer—helpful when deciding if you need a doctor. Take a Fahrenheit thermometer if possible. Otherwise convert, 37° C = 98.6° F, 39° C = 102.2° F. At the higher temperature, call a doctor.

Plastic drinking glass and spoon—they come in handy for taking medication.

**Medic Alert Precaution.** Medic Alert is a necklace or bracelet worn to let others know about your medical problems when you aren't able to tell them. On one side is an emblem recognized all over the world, while the other side describes your major illness. It also gives a telephone number stating that anyone can call it collect from any place at any time to get all pertinent data regarding your medical condition. You also receive a card to carry in your wallet with additional personal medical information. For a $15 lifetime membership, call 800-344-3226 or write Medic Alert Foundation, P.O. Box 1009, Turlock, California 95381.

**Suggestions for Diabetics.** If you should be a diabetic, Squibb & Sons Pharmaceutical Company has published an excellent brochure entitled *Vacationing With Diabetes*, which can be obtained from E. R. Squibb & Sons, Inc., World Headquarters, P.O. Box 4000, Princeton, New Jersey 08540. Among this handy booklet's suggestions is that you pack enough of your own medication, although it lists available counterparts in other countries. Those on long-active insulin should take along a bottle of regular insulin for emergencies. Since only U-40 insulin and syringes are available in many countries, it is suggested that if you are a U-80 or U-100 user, make sure to have a full supply. However, if you find that you must buy insulin abroad, conversion can be done accordingly. Multiply your usual dosage of U-80 insulin by two or a usual U-100 dosage by two-and-a-half, to determine the equivalent amount of U-40 dosages.

Squibb suggests, since dining late is frequent in many countries, that diabetics might want to take either less insulin in the morning, a second injection before going to bed, or take the usual morning dosage and have an early evening snack that contains the major part of your carbohydrate allowance for the evening. Check this with your own doctor. When sightseeing, take less insulin than usual because exercise will use up some of the ingested carbohydrates. If you should become ill on your trip, check your urine four times per day for sugar and acetone. If the tests are negative and you are vomiting, take one half of your usual insulin doses. But, if your tests show sugar, take your full dose of insulin and liquid carbohydrates (e.g. orange juice) every hour.

In case of insulin reaction, take either of the following: half a coke, three ounces of orange juice, two lumps of sugar, six or seven Lifesaver candies, or two teaspoons of honey. To prevent a second insular reaction after taking the sugar, follow with peanut butter or cheese and crackers.

Insulin lasts three months and does not have to be refrigerated but must not be left in a trunk of a car or in the sun.

***Traveling with a Pacemaker.*** It is important to have your pacemaker checked at least once a month before you leave to see if your batteries will last for the entire trip. Make sure to carry two copies of a card listing the manufacturer style, model number, type of electrode and date of implantation. It is also wise for you to avoid traveling at altitudes over 5,000 feet.

***Looking for a Doctor when Traveling.*** It's not hard to find a doctor in another country or city. Ask at the desk in your hotel. The U.S. consulate also has a list of English speaking doctors. Look in the telephone book or ask the operator to assist you.

As a precaution, you may wish to become a member of Intermedic, which provides an international directory of English speaking doctors. The directory includes doctors in more than 200 cities in 90 countries, all of whom have agreed on a standard fee. For more details, write Intermedic, Inc., 777 Third Avenue, New York, New York 10017. Another international health organization for travelers is the International Association of Medical Assistance to Travelers (IAMAT), 417 Center Street, Lewiston, New York 14092, (716) 754-4883. See also Medical Assistance for Travelers, p.*154*.

***Be Careful What You Eat.*** Think before you eat. Unwise eating is living dangerously. Avoid street vendors. People often drink water or use ice cubes even though they have been warned it may make them ill.

Moderate hotels often have in-house filtering systems although they are not always effective. Don't ask if the water is safe. Local people may not have any difficulty adjusting to the water because their bodies are conditioned to local bacteria. Most grocery or drug stores sell bottled water. If the seal is broken, leave it on the shelf. When you order bottled water in restaurants in some countries, they will give you the remainder to take home with you. Don't be bashful. Ask the waiter if you may have what is left or order a bottle to take to your room. Taking bottled water or soda with you when you go sightseeing is a wise precaution.

Don't fret if you are on a diet. There are low calorie foods in every country. Watch what you eat but give yourself a treat every now and then. When weighing yourself, 45 kilos equals 100 pounds.

Some food products are safe to eat in some parts of the world, while risky to attempt in others. Let caution rule your judgments. Unpeeled fresh fruits and vegetables may give you dysentery or other uncomfortable diseases. Although these diseases are more unpleasant than serious, they could activate other health problems for you. Usually, the farther the fruit is grown from the ground, the safer it is to eat. As you might guess, bananas are the safest fruit. Avoid raw greens outside of North America or Europe. Remember, in some tropical countries, human excrement is still used for fertilizers and this can breed disease.

Ask your waiter any questions you may have about the food you are ordering. Be sure mayonnaise, pastries, cream-filled pastries, or custards have been properly prepared and stored; they are the leading cause of food poisoning. Although dairy products are safe in Europe and North America, milk should be boiled and cheeses avoided in many tropical countries. Tuberculosis and undulent fever are sometimes transmitted through dairy products.

Fish, seafood and shellfish are wonderful eating but should be freshly caught and well cooked in hot oil, steamed, poached or broiled. Since shellfish are carriers of hepatitis and intestinal diseases, they should only be eaten when fried or boiled. Raw fish is a delicacy in Japan, Peru and some other countries. It's all right to eat if it's saltwater fish, but avoid fresh-water fish which may have worm infestations.

***Health Insurance.*** Call your insurance office and see if your health insurance will cover you while you are traveling in another country. Medicare and Medicaid will not. Your identification card is necessary for hospital coverage. When I was being treated at a hospital in Aruba, the doctor's first words were not "How are you?," but "We accept Blue Cross/Blue Shield."

***Dealing with Toileting.*** Taking care of one's toilet needs can be embarrassing and difficult. Although it is easier to urinate than manage bowel movements, both are possible. It is wiser to eat and drink less during travel and to avoid eating roughage foods such as fruits, salads and cereals. It is easier if you have your largest meal when you are near an accessible bathroom. Check with your doctor about taking anti-diarrhea medicine before traveling or an all day outing.

There are many products on the market to help solve the problems caused by your disability. Don't be embarrassed to contact a surgical supply store or manufacturing firm about your needs. Since they are in business to make or sell devices to assist you, they should be sensitive and concerned. If you write for special equipment, make sure you include money for sales tax and postage. *The Itinerary*[1] travel magazine contacted over fifty manufacturers and suppliers of toilet aids. The following are options available and where you can purchase them:

*Urinals*:
Fashionable
Crescent Avenue
Rocky Hill, New Jersey 08553-0279
telephone: 609-921-2563

---

1. *The Itinerary* (a publication of Whole Person Tours, Inc.): To Aid Travelers with Physical Disabilities, P.O. Box 1084, Bayonne, New Jersey 07002 (201) 858-3400. This excellent magazine is published six times a year.

With a little practice and discretion, anyone can use a urinal during travel. A small blanket or a Sanitary Skirt Shield made by Fashionable can give you a modicum of privacy. If you sit next to the window and your companion sits in the aisle seat, your privacy is virtually insured. Your aide can then cover the urinal with a towel or bag and discreetly take it to the bathroom for emptying and cleaning. Practice before your trip and you will become quite adept at using the urinal.

*Tinkle Tube*:
Tinkle Tube Company
P.O. Box 95
Lynden, Washington 98264
or Box 1395
Qualicum Beach
BC Canada VOR 2TO.

Though difficult in confining situations, it is leakproof. A tube goes from a funnel shaped top into a disposable receptacle or urinal. A wheelchair cushion, especially helpful for women, is designed to hold the tube.

*Catheters*:
Male catheters are available in a variety of styles in surgical supply stores. Accompanying manuals should state if they ensure against leakage. These catheters can be attached to bag receptacles that are made with different holding capacities. Make sure the bags have a flutter valve to prevent backup through the tube. Female catheters are available but are often more difficult to use.

*Waterproof Pants*:
They can be totally leakproof if used correctly. However, continual use may result in a rash. These pants are great for short periods of time and emergency use. They are also handy for bowel management during travel. Various styles are on the market. One of the more convenient models is the Maddacomfort Protector Panti (available from Maddak, Inc., Pequannock, New Jersey

07740-1993, telephone: 201-694-0500). This panty is free from binding elastic as it is held together by velcro closures, is coated and sanitized to protect against mildew and fungus growth, and can be machine washed.

*Toilet Devices:*

*Seat extenders* that raise toilet seat levels about four inches are easily cleaned, portable and adaptable without additional tools or clamps (available in several models from Maddak, Inc.). They are especially helpful to those with spinal or leg disabilities and also helpful to all wheelchair users. They can be carried in a cardboard or plastic container or can be stored in one's suitcase.

*Soft bedpans* made of vinyl and filled with cotton are portable and can be easily packed (available at your surgical supply store or from Maddak, Inc.).

*Digi-Sert*, a rectal stimulator for left or right handed people is portable, balanced and easily cleaned (available from Therafin Corporation distributors). For a list of distributors, contact Therafin Corporation, 3800 South Union Avenue, Steger, Illinois 60475, telephone: 312-755-1535.

*Digi-Sert Shur Grip* is similar to the Sert but has an additional palm plate and Velcro strip fasteners for those with little hand function (available from Therafin Corporation distributors).

*Digi-Supp E-Z Reach Combo*, a suppository inserter or digital stimulator, has interchangeable probes and a molded handle with a strap for easy use (available from Therafin Corporation distributors).

*A Folding Portable Commode* can be packed in a suitcase, weighs about 13 pounds, has adjustable seat heights and deodorant discs. When opened, it measures 21 ½" x 21" x 27 ½" and when folded its dimensions are 30 ½" x 19" x 6" (available from Maddak, Inc.).

*Other Traveling Aids*:

Other equipment is available to make your trip easier. Some devices you may want to consider are:

*Traveling Bath*—although somewhat expensive, it is an inflatable bath that folds into a small travel bag, weighs only 17 pounds, and is ideal for those who have trouble getting into a standard tub or must be bathed in a prone position. It can be placed on a bed and you would roll into the deflated tub as you would when someone is making a bed on which you are lying. A blower is used to inflate the liner. An adapter and hoses can be connected to a faucet to fill the bath with water and are later used to pump water down the drain and to deflate the tub. (Available from Ability Designs, Inc., 10C Escondido Village, Stanford, California 94305, telephone: 415-857-1053.)

*Travel Shampoo Tray*—is an inflatable vinyl tube that has a drain tube to release water into a pail. (Available from Maddak, Inc. and in most surgical supply stores.)

Your health need not be an additional concern when traveling. Take proper precautions, pack the necessary items and adhere to your doctor's advice. Eating sensibly is your best insurance for good health when traveling. If you should have a problem, don't panic; help is available.

# DIFFERENT WAYS TO TRAVEL

*Air Travel.* The air travel industry is becoming increasingly sensitive to the needs of the disabled, but, as progress rests with each individual airline, there is little consistency. This means that although air travel for the disabled is definitely accessible, it is essential to confirm with your carrier that the services and facilities you require are available.

*General Rules.* When selecting a carrier or airport, remember that, while your needs as a disabled person are valid, you are only one of many passengers. Each airline and airport has the right to make policies that concern you in the name of assuring the safety of all travelers. These policies and judgments by pilots or other personnel determine the number of disabled that can be carried and the conditions under which they will be accepted. Most of these policies are sensible in concept even if somewhat tactless in expression. For example if the flight is full, the attendant may not be able to provide special service. In that instance, it is reasonable to require the disabled passenger to have an aide. Relieved of responsibility for you, many airlines will accept more disabled people at one time, which should be considered when, for example, your wheelchair team is traveling together to a competition.

Other less palatable rulings may limit the length of a disabled person's trip or require a disabled person to sit on blankets to assure fast evacuation of the aircraft in case of an emergency.

What you will be asked to do depends on your disability and planning ahead. You can eliminate unpleasant surprises by questioning your carrier in advance and notifying them of your intentions.

Every airline is different so think of it as shopping for the best deal. You're the customer and you have concerns. Don't be shy, ask!

Does the carrier have facilities to accommodate your needs? Do they serve special diets; will they permit seeing eye dogs?

Will a flight attendant be available to give assistance if needed?

If you require special services, is there a charge?

Is there a requirement that you notify the carrier within a certain time limit that you will be traveling? Most airlines ask that you give them twenty-four hours notice.

Is the bathroom accessible? Can the aisles accommodate wheelchairs, walkers, or other equipment? If you are a paraplegic and can get to the bathroom on your hands, will they permit you to do so?

What model planes does the carrier fly? Different models vary in seating arrangements and physical features offered.

Can you pre-board? Being allowed to board before other passengers can make getting settled much easier.

How soon before take-off should you be at the airport? Even non-disabled passengers are usually requested to appear an hour before departure so consider any extra time you may need when planning.

Where should you check in? While you're asking, find out where you should go if unexpected circumstances should make you late. How will your luggage be handled? Is there curbside check-in?

Does the carrier require you to wear a button or other identifier to indicate that you need assistance? This is one of those practical rulings that can be offensive to some disabled travelers so it's wise to ask.

How are you to be boarded? Methods of boarding the disabled range from enclosed cars that transport the disabled from the terminal to the plane, to being carried in the arms of an attendant.

Where will they seat you? Most airlines seat the disabled in the bulkhead to allow them more room, but, as this is the area near the bathroom, meal tray storage and bar supplies, lines and traffic make it a mixed blessing.

Will meals be served and when? If you must eat at specific times, this is important.

What is the flight number, type of plane and number of attendants?

What is the bumping or delay policy of the airline?

Does the flight have movies, and if so, what's playing? Do they charge? There's no sense in being bored.

What size and weight luggage is allowed to be checked or as carry-on?

Are you entitled to free stopovers on international travel, thus allowing you to stop in more than one city?

Does the airline provide free transportation between domestic and international destination points in the terminal?

Can you buy one ticket for unlimited travel for so many days within a country?

Check the following chart, "Services Provided for Disabled Passengers," and see what many of the major airlines offer. However, services vary and the list may become outdated. Don't be overwhelmed.

***Airport Accessibility.*** It is important for you to know the accessibility of airports through which you will travel. *Access Travel: Airports*, published free of charge, will give you detailed information about many terminals around the world. Write the Federal Aviation Administration, U.S. Department of Transportation, Washington, D.C. 20591 for this helpful brochure. The information you will receive includes:

# SERVICES PROVIDED FOR DISABLED PASSENGERS

| | Air Canada | Air France | Air India | Alitalia | American Airlines | British Airway | Delta | El Al | Eastern Airlines | Iceland Air | Saudi Arabian Airlines |
|---|---|---|---|---|---|---|---|---|---|---|---|
| Medical questionnaire and/or certification required under various conditions | | ● | | ● | ● | | ● | | | | ● |
| No formal policy—must contact for subjective policy | | | | | | | | | | | |
| Oxygen provided and/or allows special respirators | ● | ● | | | ● | | | ● | | | ● |
| Permits guide dogs in cabins | ● | ● | | ● | ● | | | ● | ● | | |
| Preboarding | ● | ● | ● | ● | ● | ● | ● | ● | ● | ● | ● |
| Special diets provided | ● | ● | | ● | | | ● | ● | | ● | |
| Special training programs/personnel | ● | ● | | | ● | | | ● | ● | | |
| Stretcher transportation: | | | | | | | | ● | | | |
|    Requires at least one aide | ● | | | ● | | | | | | | ● |
|    Extra cost | 3 Fares | | | ● | | | | | ● | | ● |
|    Requires you arrange ambulance service | | | | ● | | | | | | | ● |
| Telewriter equipment for reservations for the deaf and speech impaired | ● | | | | ● | | | | | | |
| Wheelchair Users: Provides wheelchairs for access to plane | ● | ● | ● | | ● | ● | | ● | | ● | ● |
|    Allows motorized wheelchairs | ●* | | | | | | | | | | |
|    Carries wheelchairs free of charge | ● | | | | | | | ● | | | |
|    Installs or provides special equipment | ● | | | | | | | | | | |
|    Bathroom accessibility | ** | | | | | | | | | | |
|    Designing wheelchair for travel in plane | ** | | | | | | | | | | |
| Provides all carriers with medical kits for physicians for emergencies | ● | | | | | | | | | | |
| Quota of disabled people | | ● | | ● | | | | ● | | | |
| Companion required under various conditions | | ● | | ● | ● | | | ● | | | |
| Selected seating required | | | | | ● | ● | | ● | | | |
| Offer special services | ● | | | | | | | | ● | | |

56

*Not available on all carriers
**Providing service in newly purchased carriers

# SERVICES PROVIDED FOR DISABLED PASSENGERS

| | Scandinavian Airlines System | Swiss Air | United Airlines | U.S. Air | Transworld Airlines | National Airlines | Lufthansa Airlines | Ozark Airlines | Air Portugal | South African Airways | Iberia Airlines of Spain |
|---|---|---|---|---|---|---|---|---|---|---|---|
| Medical questionnaire and/or certification required under various conditions | • | • | | | | | • | | | • | |
| No formal policy—must contact for subjective policy | • | | | | | | | | • | • | |
| Oxygen provided and/or allows special respirators | | • | • | | | | | | | | |
| Permits guide dogs in cabins | • | • | • | • | | • | • | | | | |
| Preboarding | • | • | • | • | • | • | • | • | • | • | • |
| Special diets provided | | | | | | | • | | | • | |
| Special training programs/personnel | | | • | | | | | | | | • |
| Stretcher transportation: | | | | | | | | | | • | |
|   Requires at least one aide | | • | | | | | • | | | • | |
|   Extra cost | | • | | | | | | | | | |
|   Requires you arrange ambulance service | | | | | | | • | | | | |
| Telewriter equipment for reservations for the deaf and speech impaired | | | • | | | | | | | | |
| Wheelchair Users:<br>  Provides wheelchairs for access to plane | | • | • | | | | • | • | | | |
|   Allows motorized wheelchairs | | • | • | | | | | | | | |
|   Carries wheelchairs free of charge | | | | • | | | | | | | |
|   Installs or provides special equipment | | • | | | | | | | | | |
|   Bathroom accessibility | | | ** | | | | | | | | |
|   Designing wheelchair for travel in plane | | | ** | | | | | | | | |
| Provides all carriers with medical kits for physicians for emergencies | | | | | | | | | | | |
| Quota of disabled people | | • | | | | • | | | | • | |
| Companion required under various conditions | • | | • | • | | • | | | | • | |
| Selected seating required | | | | | | | • | | | | |
| Offer special services | | | • | | | | | | | • | |

*Not available on all carriers
**Providing service in newly purchased carriers

*Parking*:

   Parking spaces reserved for handicapped
   Directional signing to reserved spaces
   Spaces level and at least 12 feet wide
   Spaces within 2,000 feet of the terminal entrance
   Spaces protected from weather
   Parking meters and tickets accessible to the driver
   Level or ramped path from parking to entrance

*Exterior Circulation*:

   Vehicular and passenger traffic separated
   All walkways at least five feet wide
   Stairs and ramps at all changes of level
   Handrails on all ramps and stairs
   Curb cuts at all pedestrian crossings
   All ramps at least five feet wide
   All ramp slopes 8.3 percent or less
   All ramps indicated by accessibility symbol
   All ramps protected from snow and ice
   All ramp surfaces non-slip
   Ramps over 30 feet long have level rest landings
   Ramps have level landings at turns
   Ramps have handrails on both sides

*Arrival and Departure*:

   Level vehicle loading/unloading areas close to building
      entrance
   Loading/unloading areas protected from weather

*Interior Circulation*:

   Building entrances and exits level with automatic doors
   Public areas in building accessible by level/ramped route
   Public corridors at least five feet wide and obstruction free

*Elevators*:

   Public elevators accessible on level path
   Public elevators to all floors, including garage
   Elevators at least five feet by five feet inside measurement
   Elevator door opening at least three feet wide

Elevator doors have automatic safety reopening device
Elevator controls no more than four feet from floor
Elevator controls have raised lettering

*Interior Ramps*:

At least five feet wide
Slopes 8.3 percent or less
Ramp approaches indicated by accessibility symbol
Level area at least five feet by five feet at top and bottom of
  ramps
Ramps over 30 feet long have level rest landings
Landings at turning points
Handrails on both sides

*Stairs*:

Ramp or elevator available as alternate to stairs or escalators
Stairways free of projecting noses
Stairway riser height seven inches or less
Handrails on both sides

*Doors*:

Level passages at least five feet between adjacent doorways
Doors have clear opening of at least three feet
Thresholds level with floor
Level handles instead of knobs
Wall mounted paging phones not over three feet above the
  floor

*Boarding*:

Ramp or level loading bridges to aircraft

*Accommodations*:

Special transportation to other airport buildings
Car rental agencies which can provide hand controlled
  cars
Accessible hotel accommodations in airport complex
Vending machine controls identified with raised letters
Dining tables have at least a 29-inch clearance above the
  floor
Drinking fountains accessible to/usable by handicapped

*Restroom and Toilets*:

Accessible restrooms and toilets available
With five feet by five feet turning space
With at least one stall three feet wide
With at least one stall four feet eight inches deep
With at least one stall without swinging 32-inch door
With grab bars
With 29-inch clearance under lavatories
With mirrors, towels, etc. not over 40 inches above the
floor

*Phones*:

Phone with coin slot not over 48 inches high in each
phone bank
Phone with amplifier available in each bank of telephones
Raised lettering on telephone operating instructions
Telecommunications equipment available for deaf people

*Services*:

Brochures available on facilities for handicapped persons
Medical services available
Escort service available from airport or airlines

**Airports.** You will be traveling through at least two airports.
There are many questions that you will want answered concerning conditions in all the airports you will be using:

Who is notified that you're traveling? Will everyone along
the way be advised of your arrival and needs?
Is there long term parking for the handicapped at a
reasonable distance to the terminal?
Do buses and other transportation take you from the
parking lot into the terminal?
Is at least one airport restroom equipped for the
handicapped?
Are stall doors at least 32 inches wide and do they have
grab bars?
Are these restrooms identified by airport access symbols?
Does the airport have concession stands, bar and
restaurants, and are they wheelchair accessible?
Do they have curbside unloading?

Are water fountains accessible to wheelchair passengers?

Does the airport have vending machines?

Is the airport wheelchair accessible or is the only travel between floors stairs and escalators?

Where is the location of car rentals?

Is there at least one telephone mounted for the disabled? Where is it located?

If there is any need for assistance for emergencies, where do you go in each airport?

Are airline lobbies and departure gates accessible to wheelchairs?

When passengers are transferred to a narrower wheelchair at the door of the aircraft, are they transported free of charge?

Is there Skycap service to help within the airport? (Tip Skycaps a couple of dollars but do not tip airline personnel.)

**Additional Tidbits on Air Travel.** When selecting how you want to fly, be aware that there are different categories of flights:

*First Class* costs 30 to 50 percent more and gives you the luxuries of separate check-in counters, special waiting lounges, extra attention from airline personnel, more elaborate meals, free drinks, larger seats and extras such as slippers.

*Economy Coach* has narrow seats, average meals, charge for liquor or wines, and many more passengers to share the bathroom.

*Excursion* requires you to stay between 14 and 21 days or between 22 and 45 days.

*Standby* will not accept reservations and you will get a seat if one becomes available. This is the most unreliable and difficult way for a disabled person to travel. It's not worth the money saved.

*Group Inclusive Tour (GIT)* has a usual stay of 7 to 14 days with a minimum of 15 days advance purchase. If you cannot go, there is usually a penalty for cancelling your trip.

*Charters* run by both airlines and tour operators offer cheaper trips, charge for cancellation, and often have hidden liabilities, so ask a lot of questions and read contracts carefully.

***Getting Your Wheelchair Ready for Travel.*** You must prepare your wheelchair for the trip when it will be stored in the baggage compartment. If the chair is fully collapsible, it will go aboard easily. Many airlines will now allow motorized wheelchairs if only a dry cell or gel type battery is necessary. They usually require that wet cell batteries be removed, drained, and that terminals be well covered. Make sure you don't forget to ask the airline's policy on motorized wheelchairs.

When getting your wheelchair ready for storage, clearly mark your name and destination on a small sign or tag that will not come loose. Remove any loose parts such as cushions or bags that fit across the handles or over the arms and carry them on board. Lock the arms of your wheelchair in place and put the brake on so that you limit the possibility of damage.

Upon arrival, check your wheelchair for possible damage as soon as it is returned to you. If you have problems they must be reported to the airline before you leave the terminal to prove that damage or loss occurred while the chair was in the airline's possession. Airlines react differently to this situation. The staff in charge may ask their maintenance crew to fix your chair or lend you another until it is repaired. Other airlines are not as considerate and leave the problem in your hands. A car mechanic will often be able to repair your chair. A good homeowners policy, with additional coverage if necessary, is a wise precaution against damage to your wheelchair.

***Progress for Better Air Travel.*** Airlines are beginning to make greater efforts to accommodate our special needs. This is attributable to the efforts of travel groups like SATH, veteran's organizations, and the demands of individuals, especially Vietnam veterans. Speak up and make sure you have the same opportunities as others to travel easily. If an injustice is done to you or if an airline lacks an essential service, write and complain. If service was especially good, send a complimentary letter. Politely explain what is necessary to have a good flight. Do not expect the impossible. Airlines find it too expensive to convert most of their current carriers to wheelchair accessibility, but, with a known demand for better services, new carriers can be improved. Write the Federal Aviation Administration at the Department of Transportation in Washington, D.C. and explain the needs of the disabled. If you have the opportunity to testify at state or federal hearings, don't hestitate, testify. You don't need someone to write a speech for you. Simply explain your needs and what is important to a safe and comfortable flight. Your travel dollars are necessary to the travel industry and they must treat customers well.

***Traveling by Train.*** Trains are fast becoming a very desirable way for disabled people to travel. The United States insisted all trains be accessible by 1984, and many of the more than 55 train stations are barrier free.

Amtrak, the largest passenger service line in the United States, has an excellent brochure, "Access Amtrak," which you can request from the Office of Customer Relations, Amtrak, P.O. Box 2709, Washington, D.C. 20013. It details services by types of trains and even supplies blueprints of different cars so that you can check their accessibility for your needs.

Amtrak provides many services for disabled passengers, including special assistance and reduced fares. Disabled adult travelers may get a 25 percent discount if one way fare is at least $40 (children aged 2 through 11 get a 37 percent discount), provided you present a letter from a doctor ascertaining your disability, a card issued by an organization for the handicapped or a local, federal or state agency.

Hearing impaired passengers may use teletypewriters to call for reservations at 800-523-6590 or 800-523-5691 (in Pennsylvania, call 800-562-6960), and guide dogs are allowed to travel free in passenger cars.

Standard, battery operated wheelchairs are allowed on passenger cars but full powered and extra large wheelchairs must be transported in baggage cars which are not always available. Although Amtrak prefers you sit in a seat or in sleeper accommodations, if it is too uncomfortable for you they will allow you to sit in a standard wheelchair if there is room available.

Self-supporting oxygen systems may be used on trains but Amtrak requests you use sleeping rooms while traveling and notify them of your use of oxygen twelve hours in advance of your departure.

Conductors make sure you are aware of train stops and are available to assist boarding and departure. Sleeping cars have assigned attendants who will assist you when you press the button for service.

As with air travel, when making Amtrak reservations, call the Special Service Desk and explain your needs and ask for information. For the nationwide network of Amtrak telephone numbers, call 800-872-7245. "Access Amtrak" suggests sensible questions such as:

What is the best train for my particular situation?
What should I know about the railroad stations that I will be using during my trip?
Is there assistance available at the stations?
Are the station and platform to the train wheelchair accessible?
Is the station I'm using one of the 400 which offer wheelchairs for my use or must I bring my own?
Are the train aisles wheelchair accessible?
Will someone bring me my meals and assist me to the bathroom?
May I pre-board before other passengers?
If I am visually or hearing impaired, is there someone in the station and on the train to assist me?
May I order a special diet meal in the dining cars?

European rail travel is an inexpensive way to see Europe. However, it poses a great difficulty for disabled travelers, because, although some trains and stations are accessible, it is difficult for Americans to obtain information due to language barriers and the lack of available information.

In England, British Rail is updating its equipment and terminals but accessibility is spotty and you could be left in the lurch. *A Guide to British Rail for the Physically Handicapped,* which is available from the Central Council for the Disabled, 34 Eccleston Square, London SW1V1PA, England, lists stations in England and Scotland but lacks positive information to help you with access. Another brochure of interest is *British Railways: A Guide for Disabled People*, which can be obtained from the Royal Association for Disability and Rehabilitation (RADAR), 25 Mortimer Street, London W1N 8AB England.

Another difficulty in traveling by train in Europe is that necessary information is often not printed in English. If you wish information from Germany, you will have to find a translator for the brochure available from FKD Gesselschaft fur Medizineschen Tourismus, 8720 Schweenfurt Postfach 1245, West Germany.

If your travel agent or a friend knows people in the countries you want to visit, perhaps they could help plan your trip. For most of us, the language barriers and lack of factual data makes traveling through Europe by train impossible.

**Traveling by Bus.** If you are going to travel in the United States or Canada, investigate the possibility of traveling by bus. This is an excellent way to travel that is not only comfortable and economical but is also often the friendliest and most informal way of traveling. Many bus travelers make friends along the way since much time is spent on the bus and there is lots of opportunity for conversations. Since buses travel through cities, small towns and the countryside, they afford one the opportunity to see more scenery than any other form of public transportation. (Contact: Helping Hand Service for the Handicapped, Greyhound Lines, Greyhound Towers, Phoenix, Arizona 85077.)

The two major bus companies, Greyhound and Trailways, offer special incentives for you:

You and a traveling companion may ride for the price of one adult fare if you have a written statement from your doctor that you need physical assistance.

Non-motorized wheelchairs and many other aids are carried free of charge.

If you travel without a companion, personnel will meet

you at the curb and take you to the bus if you call and make arrangements in advance.

You will be pre-boarded and have a choice of the front seats.

Buses are temperature controlled for your convenience in any weather.

Food is available at Greyhound terminals or at frequent rest stops, or it is quite common to bring your own.

If you need your wheelchair at rest stops, the driver will unload it for you.

The bus companies will help you find hotels, motels and restaurants near their terminals if you have to stay overnight on your trip.

Greyhound offers Ameripass which allows unlimited travel in the United States over a period of time depending on the price of the ticket you buy. You may purchase one for 7, 15 or 30 days.

Greyhound and Trailways have attempted to make their terminals more accessible by providing wider doorways, handrails, ramps, convenient restrooms, and, in some places, telephones at wheelchair level. However, they have hundreds of terminals and many have not been improved.

Call the bus companies and ask for staff from Greyhound's "Helping Hand Service" or Trailways' "Good Samaritan Plan" and tell them where and when you want to travel. Ask about the accessibility of terminals. Explain your need for accessible accommodations if you must stay overnight on your trip, and let them know you will need assistance when it is necessary to transfer from bus to bus or in different terminals.

***Travel by Car.*** Traveling by car is the most personal way to take a trip. You make all the decisions about when and where you will go. Like buses, cars allow you to travel various routes and afford you the opportunity of choosing a wide menu of places to see. Car travel also allows you the most freedom in making accommodations to your personal health conditions. If you find you are more tired than expected, stay an extra day. If you find you have a surge of energy, adjust your schedule once again.

***Travel in the United States.*** It's not difficult to plan trips in the United States. Write to states, cities or places of interest, using addresses in access books (see Access Information, p.*99*). Gather maps and check routes. Perhaps you wish to have AAA map your journey. Many restaurants along the way are accessible to you. A brochure, *Highway Rest Areas for Handicapped Travelers*, is available from the President's Committee on Employment of the Handicapped, Washington, D.C. 20210, which lists by state and specific locations those rest areas with facilities to accommodate disabled travelers.

***Traveling Abroad by Car.*** Once you get to another country, you will find that traveling by car has decided advantages. You become free of timetables, reservations and set itineraries. Since you have more freedom to choose different travel routes, it opens up opportunities to explore out of the way places. In Europe, cars are also an inexpensive way to travel since towns and cities are not too far apart.

The disadvantages of auto travel include congested traffic and limited parking in many cities. Poor and unmarked roads can make driving more difficult. Good maps are essential while a good sense of direction is a decided advantage.

A good way to estimate travel time is to limit yourself to 100 miles or 170 kilometers without a rest. Plan an extra hour or two for unfamiliar, winding or poor roads. Allow a lot of extra time at ferry crossings for the wait.

Renting cars abroad can be done by your travel agent at home. Every major airport, train terminal or pier has either AAA, Hertz, Avis or Auto Europe. Prices fluctuate according to country and season. You can either rent a car by the day and pay additionally for each mile traveled, or you can pay a larger flat fee regardless of how far you travel. Some details to consider when renting a car are:

Reserve four weeks in advance and get a written
confirmation.
Make sure the height and width of the car can easily

accommodate you and your wheelchair, if necessary.

If you rent through a travel agent, make sure you have in writing the type of car you ordered, dates needed, and all conditions of payment including charges for mileage, gas or leaving the car in another country.

Make sure you carefully read an English version of the contract before you sign it. Beware of the fine print that may state prices are subject to change.

Request automatic or standard shift ahead of time. Some agencies will rent you a car with special controls for the disabled traveler. In the United States, Avis (800-331-1212), Hertz (800-654-3131) and National Car Rentals (800-328-4567) will have some hand controlled cars for no extra charge at some places. Also check Disabled Drivers Association, Ashwellthorpe Hall, Ashwellthorpe, Norwich NOR 89W, England; Handicapped Drivers Mobility Guide, American Automobile Association, 811 Gatehouse Road, Falls Church, Virginia 22042; and Auto Europe, 25 West 58th Street, New York, New York 10019.

Other places that rent hand controlled cars are:

Paris
Inter-Touring Service
117 Boulevard August, Blangurl/ 7501 Paris, France.

England
Kening Car Hire Ltd.
447-479 Green Lane, Palmers Green/ London N13, England.

Ireland
Kenning Car Hire Ltd.
42-43 Westland Road/ Dublin 2, Ireland.

Australia
Letz Rent a Car/ Australian Tourist
1270 Avenue of the Americas/ New York, New York 10020.

Check a nation's rental policies since some have rules that limit rentals. In England, you must be between 21 and 65 to rent a car.

Many car rental agencies insist on credit card ownership before they will rent to you so they will have a way to bill you if the car is damaged or not returned.

If you cancel reservations far enough in advance you often get a full refund. However, if you decide you don't want to rent a car after the cancellation date stated, you probably will have to pay a penalty fee. If you return the car in fewer days than you paid for, most rental agreements will insist that you pay for the full time period. Some companies will refund part of your money and charge a cancellation fee. There are usually fees required for returning a car late.

Usually the car rental company is responsible for repairs required when you are on the road. You must put out the money and they will reimburse you. However, if it will cost more than $50, you should call the rental dealer and see if they will authorize the additional costs. Keep all bills and receipts for reimbursement.

Some tips for driving abroad are:

Driver's licenses are usually accepted from over-18 drivers, but some nations prefer you have the AAA's International Driving Permit. This one year permit will cost you $5 and requires presentation of your driver's license and two passport size photos for issuance.

Some countries require registration papers to prove ownership when you are traveling through more than one country. They may be obtained from sales agents at the time of car purchase.

Many European countries require you to purchase a "Green Card" for insurance purposes. Both rental and sales agents will arrrange for coverage.

Gasoline, called petrol, essence, benzina or Benzin, will be more expensive than prices you are used to in the United States. However, within the United States, it will vary according to the section of the country in which you are traveling.

When you buy gas, ten liters is approximately 3 gallons (see Metric Conversion Tables, p 128 ). One kilometer equals .6 miles and ten kilometers are just over 6 miles, so to compute mileage, just multiply kilometers.

In Great Britain, the Virgin Islands, and some other countries, cars travel on the left side of the road. To cut down on hazards from this unfamiliar driving pattern, avoid rush hours in crowded areas, don't drive when tired or in pain, and, in general, be more alert.

Make sure your car is locked at all times and store luggage and valuables in the trunk whenever possible to discourage theft. Unfortunately, rented cars with special license plates are invitations to local thieves.

When planning your travel itinerary, make sure you know when local holidays and festivals are or you may find that you unwillingly can only travel at a slow pace because of local events. Your travel agent or national tourist offices will give you this information. You may also wish to arrange your trip to attend one of these local fiestas. Traveling by car allows this greater opportunity for seeing more local color and how people in a country really live.

Buying a foreign car, using it for travel, and then shipping it to the United States has both advantages and disadvantages. The pluses are that you will have a convenient vehicle that should meet all your needs for a lower price than you would pay at home, since you will not pay for foreign import taxes, and car dealers in various countries may set lower prices to encourage purchase by tourists. You will also pay a lower U.S. duty charge since the car will be used and not new when it enters the United States. The minuses of buying a car in another country and shipping it home may include the lack of American anti-pollution devices (which are costly to add afterwards), time-consuming shopping and bureaucratic red tape involved in a major purchase in a foreign country, pre-duty and inspection charges required in some countries, and special marine insurance when it is shipped home.

Consider all the pros and cons of auto travel and decide if it appeals to you. If you want to drive, carefully make plans to rent or buy your car (see Different Ways to Travel, p.66). A travel agent can be helpful in implementing your plans.

*Cruises.* The cruise industry has made great strides in recent years in making cruise travel more comfortable for the disabled. Cruise staff give outstanding service. They are attentive, responsive and reliable. Many special cruises have been arranged to serve particular disabilities.

I have found, however, that cruises are difficult for disabled people. It took me many years to get up the courage to try a cruise. It was even tougher than I imagined. The cabins are usually not built for wheelchairs. Often there are one or two steps which make travel harder. Doorways are narrow and difficult to keep open. Ships, rocking with the waves, often make wheelchairs tip or slide and walking may be precarious even for healthy people. Elevators are small and crowded. Cruises are certainly a challenge to be carefully considered according to your disability.

*Subways.* Although it is almost impossible to travel on most subways, the Metro in Washington, D.C., which has stations conveniently located at points of interest, accommodates the disabled traveler whether he or she is blind, deaf or wheelchair bound. Its clearly marked access elevators at all stations are large, well lit and equipped with rails, safety mirrors and brailled signals. Computerized fare cards are sold from machines located near elevators. Subway cars, which are clean and air conditioned, have designated seating for the disabled and designated spaces with poles for support of wheelchair travelers. Platforms and subway cars are of equal height for smooth wheelchair and visually impaired access.

# WHEN YOU GET THERE

There is a variety of information that will make your trip easier for you once you arrive at your destination. This potpourri of information is indexed for your convenience:

***Arrival.*** Relax and be patient. You will probably be asked to wait until everyone else has debarked and the aisles are clear. This has advantages because, while other passengers are standing and waiting, you'll be comfortable. Another plus for waiting is that you won't have to wait for your luggage. By the time you're ready, so is your baggage.

When it is your turn, someone from the airline will be there to assist you to the baggage claim area. If you're traveling abroad you will have to pass through customs after claiming your luggage. Most countries allow certain items to be brought in duty-free, including reasonable amounts of new clothing, radios, camera equipment, typewriters, film and cigarettes. If you have questions about these items, call or write the local consulate of the country you will be visiting, or ask your travel agent. During customs inspection you may be asked where you are staying and for how long. If the country requires a passport, it will be stamped and you will be allowed to enter (see Visas and Passports, p.*160*).

***Leaving the Airport.*** If you plan to rent a car, do so before you leave home. That way it will be waiting and you need only ask where the rental desk of your specific rental service is located. Taxis, cabs, limousines and airport buses are usually located directly outside the terminal. Limousines or airport bus service between the airport and specific hotels is usually cheaper than a taxicab but will take longer because buses usually stop at several hotels. Be sure to ask the number to call to arrange for your return trip to the airport. Twenty-four hours prior to leaving, confirm your flight and then call the limousine or bus service and ask when and where you will be picked up. If possible, check with your travel agent before you leave and see if the round trip from airport to hotel can be arranged in advance. It may be that the cost of this transportation is included in the cost of your trip.

***Go Directly to Your Hotel.*** Although you may be anxious to explore your new surroundings, hold off. Take a nap. Give your body a chance to recover from jet lag and time changes. Taking care of yourself now ensures a healthier trip later on. If you are too excited to sleep, rest and plan some of your next day's events. Ask the hotel for brochures and information about local tours and special events. Inquire if there is a nearby bookstore or gift shop: you may want to see if they have any books on the local area. If you must venture out, the beginning of your trip is a good time to buy theater tickets in advance. Heeding this advice, I purchased the last two tickets and saw Rudolf Nureyev dance. Had I waited, I would have missed the opportunity because the performance was sold out.

***Hotels.*** Although you may have investigated the facilities of your hotel in advance, if the accommodations are inconvenient for you, don't hesitate to ask the clerk to help find ones that fit your needs. If that fails, call the consulate or even ask a stranger who speaks English to help you. Don't be shy.

In judging your accommodations, keep in mind that you are not at home. Europe or Africa is not the United States. You went abroad for new sights and different ways and you must expect things to be new and different. For example, there may be no soap provided, so take your own just in case. The most common difference you may observe is in the toilet facilities or water closets. Men and women often use the same bathrooms. Stalls do not reach the floor, so don't be surprised to see the feet of someone of the opposite sex in the next stall. Many countries also have fixtures that look like low toilets. These are called bidets and are used to wash the genitals. The proper way to use them is a mystery to most Americans so don't worry about it.

The use of water may vary depending on where you are visiting. In the tropics, there may be a restriction on the amount of water you can use. If this is the case, the hotel will notify you. I encountered a restriction on water use when I visited England during a drought, most unusual for that country. Speaking of water, it's important to know the words for hot and cold to avoid accidents in the bathroom. Hot is *caliente* in Spanish, *chaude* in French and *hess* in German. Cold is *frio* in Spanish, *froide* in French and *kalt* in German. Check a dictionary and learn these terms in the language of each of the countries you will be visiting.

Some countries have unusual sleeping arrangements. In Japan, some hotels supply sleeping mats instead of beds. If it is at all possible, try and experiment with different local customs. However, if your disability prohibits experimentation, look for other accommodations.

A plus that is often available at hotels abroad and less frequently in the United States, is the concierge, or hotel help extra-ordinaire. Their purpose is to solve the guests' problems, regardless of size. They can help plan trips, give directions to wherever you may wish to go, buy theater tickets, and advise you where to get stamps and mail letters. You can contact this extremely useful person through the hotel desk, travel desk or bell captain.

Hotel lobbies are wonderful for disabled travelers. They serve as a place to observe other travelers, meet people, and, often, drink and relax. It's the safest place to make contact with others because if someone should prove disagreeable or a nuisance, there are people around to come to your rescue.

I never travel without cards or a backgammon set. If I bring them to the lobby at night, someone invariably offers to play with me. Also, it allows my companion to go out without me.

Many hotels have a library. In Switzerland I found that hotels not only had libraries but game rooms and movies for guests. All in all, your hotel can be much more than just a place to sleep.

If you still have time on your hands in the evening you can help yourself and others by keeping a diary. For you, it will be a record for the future. For others, especially the disabled, it will be a record of the pros and cons of where you have been: accessibility, restaurants, local tourist attractions, and good places to shop. Another evening chore that can make traveling easier is counting your foreign currency and making sure you have enough money. Banks are the cheapest and best places to exchange money, but it can be done in your hotel if it is more convenient for you. Be aware that hotels usually add on a 20 to 40 percent service charge, and exchanging money in restaurants or stores is even more expensive. Plan ahead and save money.

***Checking Out.*** Before you leave your hotel, carefully check your room since it is difficult to reclaim items after checking out. If you packed on an unmade bed, check between the sheets for a lost item, especially something the same color as the sheets. Look under your pillows, since, in some European countries, maids will put your bed clothes there. Look under the bed for slippers, shoes, cane tips and anything else you may have dropped. Check shelves for cameras, pocketbooks or gifts, and don't forget gifts or valuables that you may have hidden in your room. Recheck medicine cabinets and behind bathroom doors for sundry bathroom items that are easily forgotten. Make sure you haven't sent anything to the cleaners or laundry that you forgot to pick up. Remember to remove all valuables from the hotel safe and to pick up your passport if you were required to leave it at the hotel desk.

***Hairdressers.*** Having your hair done professionally is a luxury for some and a necessity for other disabled people. If your hotel has a beauty shop, patronize it because it will be easier to reach, it is usually more reliable and the hairdressers will be more likely to speak English. If you enjoy having your hair done, make time in your schedule. Hairdressers are tipped the same as you would at home.

***Telephones.*** It is more difficult to telephone in a foreign country than it is at home. First there may be a language barrier, and, second, you may need a token. The easiest way to make a telephone call is through the hotel operator who is used to making calls for foreign travelers.

With public telephones, find out before you make a call if you have to go somewhere to buy a token. Make the telephone call as you would in a public booth in the United States. Often you can hear the person when they answer, but, until you release the lever which releases the token, the person can't hear you.

***Dealing with Differences.*** Although we travel to visit someplace different, we sometimes expect the people and customs to be the same as at home or as we imagine them from the movies. It's best to just bring an open mind. Many of your preconceptions may be as incorrect as those of the visitor to the United States who expects to see cowboys and gangsters. Respect and enjoy the differences in the places you travel. Also, since you may be the only person from your country others meet, be a goodwill ambassador.

English is spoken as a second language in most countries, but you will be a welcome guest if you attempt to speak the native language. Your accent and even your mistakes will endear you to them. Be brave, be bilingual.

Aside from the language, you will have to deal with many other differences. Even simple foods can change around the world. In many European and South American countries, coffee is much stronger than we are accustomed to drinking. If you dislike strong coffee, take coffee bags or decaffeinated coffee from home. You can use a heating coil to prepare coffee in your room and it is perfectly proper to ask your waiter to bring you a cup of hot water in a restaurant.

Local customs relating to time and how it is perceived can complicate your life. In some places, people are not as concerned with time as we are, and their pace is different. Promptness may not be a priority. In Spain, Mexico, South America and many island countries, the leisurely pace is most relaxing. If you are inconvenienced, be patient. You will be amazed at how easy it is to accept throwing away the clock. Besides, slowing down is good for your health. Try to adjust to local timetables. Often people in countries that pride themselves on their fine cuisine, such as France and Italy, dine later in the evening. Latin and South American restaurants are open until the wee hours of the morning while, in England, dinner is eaten much earlier than in the United States. Don't forget, however, that dietary habits associated with your health and medications should be adhered to carefully. Eat a snack if you become hungry or require it when taking medicine.

**Sightseeing.** The best way to enjoy the differences of traveling is to approach sightseeing in a systematic manner. Knowledgeable sightseers have the most successful trips. Consult travel books and brochures. Question tour guides. Ask at the hotel desk, U.S. consulate or talk to local people. Find out when stores, restaurants, banks, and tourist sites are open. Inquire about customs which may affect scheduling, such as the siesta, where many businesses close down during an afternoon nap period. Traveling during major religious holidays or sabbaths may also affect planning.

It is wise to keep the spirit of religious worshippers or countries and behave as they do on their day of worship.

Although the sabbath is Sunday in most Christian countries of Europe and South America, it is Friday in Moslem countries and, in Israel, it is observed from sundown on Friday until sundown on Saturday. Don't plan sightseeing tours unless you investigate because, on the sabbath in many countries, streets are empty and stores and buildings are closed. Days of worship, when most things are closed, are good days to leave to whim. I especially like to visit Hyde Park in London on Sundays when speakers stand on their boxes and expound their different theories. In some countries, Sunday afternoons are the day for spectator sports such as bullfights and soccer games.

Easter weekend in Canada is celebrated from Friday through Monday and many places are closed. Holidays can also mean lost time due to increased traffic and numbers of tourists. In Italy, I avoided Rome between Good Friday and Easter Sunday and used the three days to visit Florence, where I saw beautiful but lesser known special Easter festivities at the cathedral, with its spectacular fireworks display.

Organized sightseeing provides the best results. Begin by investigating a new city on a bus tour or, if you meet other travelers, ask them to share a taxi trip with you. I found taxi trips to be cheaper and more personalized, and they provide the opportunity to share an overview of a city. An initial survey will give you a sense of direction and an idea of the sights you wish to explore further. Budget sightseeing time by planning to visit places in only one section of the city or country rather than wasting time and effort making haphazard choices.

Access to tourist sites is contantly changing. When I first visited Hawaii, the Pearl Harbor Memorial provided some services for the disabled, but it was impossible to board the Arizona Memorial in the middle of the harbor. Returning six weeks later, I was pleasantly surprised to find newly installed ramps that made the entire site available to me. If you really want to see a place you read was not accessible, call and check to see if improvements have been made.

Although you may have planned to the best of your ability, be prepared to alter your agenda. You may discover new places of interest at any time. One rainy day in Copenhagen, when we had to cancel a boat trip, the desk clerk recommended a tour of the Carling Brewery. Even though I could not participate in part of the tour because of access limitation, I had a wonderful time. I joined the other tourists in the banquet room where tables were set with flags from the countries of that day's guests. While testing free beer and soda, I had an opportunity to socialize, learn about places to visit and good restaurants, and also to hear news from home. In London, during a drought, I changed my plans in the opposite direction. Making the most of the sunshine, which is unusual in the British Isles, I put aside visits to indoor museums and galleries for another trip.

***Shopping*** Some folks like to spend a good part of their vacations shopping while others want to spend as little time as possible buying gifts and souvenirs. If traveling with a companion, decide before you leave home how much time will be spent shopping in order to avoid conflicts.

Europe no longer has the bargains that were once so desirable to American travelers. However, that doesn't mean that certain items aren't reasonable and often cheaper than back home. In Europe, one may shop in the many specialty stores, auction houses, small antique stores, boutiques and outdoor markets and stores and find items not available at home for any price. In some cities, certain streets are noted for their specialty shops, like Carnaby Street in London displaying the latest in fashion.

Department stores are convenient places to shop since they have the advantage of a wide array of merchandise, easy shipment home, delivery to hotels, and acceptance of major credit cards. Harrods in London sells clothes, foods, gifts, furniture, appliances, antiques, provides trip planning and offers one of the best "teas" in town.

The dollar and its value often determines if you will get a bargain. If the rate of exchange for American money is high you will find that you will get much more for your money. The truest bargains are usually found for items that are manufactured within the country since there is little cost for shipping and duties.

While planning your trip it is wise to learn where products are made in the countries you will visit. This extra research often clues you in on the best places to buy goods in a country. When traveling the Greek Islands, it is smart to buy what you can in Rhodes since it has a tax agreement with the government and can sell its goods more cheaply. Usually, souvenirs of one's trip are treasured more if they truly represent the country in which you traveled.

Strolling through foreign markets gives you the opportunity to browse or buy when ordinarily, at home, you wouldn't have the time. I cherish a wood carving purchased on a trip to Canada many years ago. I knew it wasn't a bargain but it was beautiful and, for all my years of pleasure, has been well worth the money spent.

Purchasing clothes in foreign countries can prove difficult. In the United States sizes are measured by inches while in Europe and in Latin American countries they are measured in centimeters. A good rule of thumb is 2 ½ centimeters to every inch. (See Clothing Sizes, p. *159*, for comparable sizes.) These charts are approximations so try on clothes whenever possible. If you are purchasing clothes for a gift, ask a sales clerk or another shopper who appears to be the right size to try it on for you. They usually don't mind. If in doubt, buy something a little larger so it can be taken in if necessary.

Check the fabric and how the clothes are made. Russia sells beautiful furs but they are often badly processed and wear poorly. If you can anticipate what you will be shopping for, check prices before you leave home so you will know if the clothing you are purchasing is really a bargain.

There are many books available for antique shoppers working their way through European stores and auctions. Dealers often travel to Europe to buy for their shops. Although London is still the auction capital of the world, Copenhagen, Paris, Rome, Brussels, Vienna, Munich and Zurich also have fine antiques. Amateur collectors are welcome to attend auctions.

Research may substitute for experience. Beware of phony antiques and furniture by carefully examining everything you buy. Defects and imitations are common.

European open markets are great fun even if they no longer offer the bargains they once did. Here are some suggestions to help you wind you way through the many stalls, stands and stores:

- Find out from the hotel desk or concierge what days and hours the outdoor markets are open and ask about local customs regarding haggling. Most markets open at seven in the morning and close at noon.
- Haggling is an art in which the buyer and seller come together on a price—but only after each has had his say. You may not get the biggest bargain but you'll have fun. In haggling, it is expected that you will disagree with the shopkeeper on the price. You will be respected if you take the time and thought to do it in style. Learn to say "too expensive" in the native language. Remember both you and the seller have roles to play. You may walk away threatening not to buy, he may feign ignorance of English to confuse you. You may challenge the price and discreetly imply the goods aren't worth the price. Obviously, a bit of poker player's deadpan is an asset. Wear inexpensive clothing and little jewelry; if they think you can afford more, they will charge it. It's a game and you may be the winner.
- The best times to shop for a bargain are when it's cold and rainy or at the end of the day when the seller is anxious to go home. These bargains may only cost you inconvenience and cold feet.
- When evaluating if you have a true bargain, add in the cost of shipping the item home.
- Beware of pickpockets. Hide your money in several places, including hard to reach spots such as underwear.
- Wear comfortable shoes when walking. Those in wheelchairs have a definite advantage for these excursions.
- Only buy items that you will use when you get home. It is so tempting to buy a sombrero or other colorful items but

think about what you will do with it afterwards. You will be the most unpopular person if you decide to give these useless items as Christmas or birthday presents. Some excellent buys are gold jewelry and leather items in Florence, Italy and beautiful handmade sweaters from Ireland, Iceland or the Scandinavian countries. These home produced goods are cheaper than when purchased in the United States, so be well informed for successful shopping.

Duty-free shops have sprung up around the world in airports, resort towns and cities. While they once held many bargains, this is no longer true. Often the difference in the rate of exchange has diminished the opportunities for bargains. Discount shopping at home is often the best buy you can find. The price includes shipping costs and allows you to return things when they don't live up to expectations.

Even with all the precautions, don't be discouraged from bringing home gifts for yourself and others. You will cherish them as reminders of your trip. Carefully choose what you buy and don't get caught up in a false euphoria of great bargains.

*Eating.* Once again, remember you are not at home. Even if you are on a diet, there are many new things you can try in every country. You may not like some things after tasting them but be brave and at least try. I was shocked to discover that a delicious dish I ordered was, in fact, raw squid. I am glad that I sampled first and found out later. It was wonderful.

There are, of course, some rules for sensible eating. Abide by the advice in the Health Section of this book. Dr. Hayes is sensible when she cautions against certain foods. "Montezuma's Revenge" and its variations in other countries come from ignoring a few precautionary measures. Don't overdo it with too much rich food and wine. Not only may you feel ill, it may make you sluggish.

Remember you don't have to eat in restaurants all the time. Purchasing food in local stores saves money and can be fun. A loaf of bread, cheese, fruit and wine make a great picnic.

If you're going to a restaurant, there are things to know that can save you money. Sometimes highly touted restaurants found in travel books and hotel directories may be tourist traps featuring higher prices and lower quality in exchange for "ambiance." A better value in most cases is the tourist price dinner available in restaurants all over Europe. The menu varies each day and the cost is about one third of the regular dinner. While traveling in Scandinavia, we ate these meals every night and enjoyed them immensely. They had the added advantage of not allowing one to get in a rut and they widened my gourmet horizons. To find a good restaurant, local advice is still my favorite method. Carry translations of words for food with you. Drink local wines and beers; they are cheaper and often superior since they are local specialties. In Scandinavia, the drink is schnapps with a beer chaser. Make sure, however, that you have checked with your doctor or pharmacists to assure against possible drug interactions.

**Tipping.** Tipping policy varies in different countries, but, in general, a waiter should get between fifteen and twenty percent. If the captain has prepared a salad or special dessert, he should get five percent. The maître d' who performs a special service such as arranging a special table or getting you a table when they are all reserved should get five to ten dollars. The wine steward receives four to ten dollars depending on the amount of time he has spent assisting you. In some countries the tip is included in the bill. In Russia, tipping in restaurants is forbidden by the government but checkrooms expect a tip for handling your hat and coat. In China, tipping is considered insulting. Avoid embarrassment and check local tipping customs with guides or at your hotel.

A rule of thumb for hotels is at least twenty-five cents per suitcase with a fifty cents minimum. In large cities, the minimum should be one dollar. Chambermaids usually receive one dollar per day or five dollars per week. As in restaurants, local practices and customs may affect tipping in hotels. In some countries, such as Portugal, tips are included in the room cost as a service charge.

The smartest course of action is to inquire beforehand to

assure that your gratuity is appropriate. Aside from the possiblity of offending by undertipping, a traveler may do himself a disservice by overtipping. Although customs vary from country to country, where tipping is permitted, those who make life easier for the disabled deserve generous treatment. When in Egypt, I met a bell captain who called a taxi and negotiated a price, saving me from being overcharged. He also made sure the driver would honor the agreement by advising me to pay part of the fee when I reached the Sphinx and the rest when I was safely back at the hotel.

Another example of someone who deserved and received more consideration was the desk clerk in a small town in Switzerland that had no taxi service. He arranged for a car and a driver at my disposal. Finally, I would be remiss if I didn't mention England, where I found the people especially gracious. The taxis were wide and the drivers outstanding for their courtesy and attentiveness. I found that I tipped most heavily there and I was glad I brought additional money.

Other situations where tipping is questionable are chartered tours and with officials. Tour passengers usually contribute a share and tip the guides and drivers at the end of the trip, but some tours include such tips in the cost of the ticket so check when you sign up. Never attempt to tip a customs or immigration official. Your gratitude may be misunderstood and they may suspect you are trying to bribe them.

A general observation on tipping is, you should pay for what you get. Disabled travelers need extra service. Where it is offered we should recognize that our needs are more than usual and be willing and happy to pay for it.

*Photography.* Taking pictures of your trip is important not only for the memories that they evoke; they are also a reminder of what you can accomplish. Camera equipment today is simple to operate—instamatics, discs, auto-focus, and pre-set 35mm cameras. Even if you can't manipulate a camera, take one along and ask a fellow traveler or tour guide to take your picture and you will find they are more than happy to oblige. If you don't want to bother taking snapshots or want to supplement your collection with more professional pictures, buy postcards throughout your trip.

Special equipment designed to assist disabled photographers includes shoulder pads to hold your camera, tripods set on a lapboard to give wheelchair photographers greater control, and a camera with a cable release held in your mouth to move the shutter.

If you have a new camera, use a roll of film at home in as many different conditions as you can imagine to become familiar with the camera and also ensure that it is working properly. Read a good book on photography to find out about light and the best way to photograph your subjects.

Buy your film at home since it is much more expensive in other countries. Be generous with the amount you buy. It is easy to return when you get home because all film carries at least a two-year expiration date, but aside from the cost, you may not be able to buy extra film that is just what you need in a small town in another country. Also be sure to carry extra batteries; some of the new auto-wind cameras use a new battery every four or five rolls of film.

To make sure that airport x-ray machines do not spoil your film, buy a lead or steel bag in a photography store. This small investment usually holds about ten rolls of film. In airports and throughout your travels keep your camera with you at all times. Don't put it on the back of your chair in a restaurant or lay it down haphazardly on a sightseeing bus where it can be easily stolen.

Be a polite photographer. Don't hold up tours to take one more picture. Some people dislike being subjects for tourists' pictures so ask their permission first. In some cultures, like the Amish in Pennsylvania, it is against peoples' religion to be photographed. In some parts of the world, natives want rewards for being photographed. Adults will usually ask for money and children often prefer gum or candy. Don't forget to occasionally ask someone to photograph you in front of a famous site so your pictures will show that you were there.

# WHAT IF DISASTER STRIKES?

***Disasters Do Occur.*** Unfortunate incidents do happen and it makes sense to take preventive measures to cut down on the possibilities of mishaps. You may be the unlucky person who has something stolen or whose baggage is lost. The best way to handle these potential situations is described in the next sections.

***Protect Your Home Before You Leave.*** You will feel more secure about leaving your home if you make an effort to protect it before you leave. Make your home look as if someone is still living in it. Alert your neighbors that you will be away and ask them to periodically check your house and to call the police if they should see anything suspicious.

Since accumulations of mail are obvious evidence of your absence, ask a friend or neighbor to collect your mail daily, have the doorman or superintendent of your apartment building hold your mail, or ask the local post office to hold your mail by writing a letter specifying your dates of departure and return. In a large city, a driver's license or passport will help you identify yourself when you claim your mail; in a small town, the mail carrier will probably deliver your mail when you request it.

Perhaps this is the time to purchase the alarm system that you thought was a sound precaution, but never bothered to install. There are electronic alarms that ring very loudly if someone enters your house and alarms that connect directly to a police station. If you should install one of these devices and then have someone check your house while you are away, make sure you inform that person how to prevent the alarm from going off.

Another good precaution is hooking up inexpensive timers to lamps so that they will go on and off every day as if someone were occupying the house. Some people prefer to have a friend, relative or student move into their house when they are gone to provide maximum protection and to care for pets and plants.

It is wise to put your valuable jewelry and silver pieces in a safe deposit box at your local bank. This is an inexpensive way to guarantee that your valuables will be secure. Put sentimental pieces that mean a great deal to you regardless of their material value in a safe place as well.

*If Someone Needs to Locate You.* Although it may be difficult, it is not impossible for someone from home to locate you if an emergency should arise. Leave your itinerary with the dates you will be at each hotel with the hotel telephone numbers (if possible), with an appropriate person that others might contact if there is an emergency. If you can't be reached at a hotel, an American consulate can contact local police, hotels and hospitals, if necessary. However, calling an American consulate makes for a precarious search at best. It often depends on the emergency, who is reached at the consulate, and how much work is pressuring the consulate when they are notified. Also, the Privacy Act of 1974 states that you must give written permission to the local consulate if you wish to be contacted, otherwise they cannot reach you unless your health or safety is jeopardized. It is best to let the American consulate in each country know where you will be staying if you want to be available for emergencies at home.

*Your Flight Has Been Delayed or Cancelled.* Flight delays are annoying, but common, occurrences. Airlines are not legally responsible for your inconvenience or the consequences of delays. If your delay is four hours or less there is not much you can do. But if you are delayed more than four hours, the airline is usually responsible for finding you another flight, providing food and lodging, and offering appropriate transportation to and from hotels and restaurants. Many large airlines offer kits with toiletries for overnight stays. Normally, small airlines don't have these services.

If your flight is delayed or cancelled, you don't have to wait to book a flight on another airline. Tickets for scheduled airlines are sometimes interchangeable among different companies. If you think an airline is continually stalling by announcing hour delays, look to another airline for a more immediate flight. However, you will probably have to pay any difference in the price of the ticket.

Each airline decides its own policies. Some airlines will only provide one meal no matter how long you are delayed. Often a free meal is a voucher for a restaurant in the airport and doesn't include alcoholic beverages.

Many flights are overbooked to ensure that the plane is completely filled. In those cases where there are more passengers than seats, someone must wait and take the next flight in a procedure called "bumping." Airlines usually ask for volunteers so don't be afraid you will be stranded. Those who are bumped receive, on a space available basis, a free round-trip ticket to any place the airline travels on its normal routes. Although getting bumped can be disrupting to your travel plans, it's a cheap way to be sure you can travel again.

***Baggage Delayed/Lost/Stolen.*** If your luggage is delayed, lost or stolen, try to treat it as an inconvenience and don't let it ruin your trip. To ensure that you are compensated, keep your baggage claim ticket to prove you checked your luggage aboard the flight. If your luggage is not available at your destination, go to the airline's luggage claim office, fill out a missing baggage report and keep a copy for yourself. It is useful to report lost or damaged luggage before you leave the airport so that there is no question that the luggage was lost or damaged during the flight. If you are not able to fill out the required form at the airport, you have twenty-one days to file a claim for lost luggage and seven days for damaged luggage. Often your luggage will follow on the next flight and you will be asked to await its arrival. Usually, lost luggage arrives within twenty-four hours. My advice for reducing the chances for lost luggage is to check the tags on the luggage after it has been checked to make sure that the airline attendant has written the correct flight number and destination on them. Incorrect tags are the cause of a lot of lost luggage.

If your luggage won't arrive for several hours, the airline usually sends it to you at their expense. If your bags are delayed and you need to purchase necessary items, most airlines are authorized to approve immediate expenditures. You will either receive cash from the airline or it will ask you to buy what you need and mail them the receipts for reimbursement. It's a good idea to check with airline personnel before you make any major purchase to see how much money they will allow you to spend. If your luggage did not arrive in time for an important meeting, you will need to buy a shirt, suit, shoes and other necessary articles of clothing, but ascertain the airline's liability before shopping.

If you never receive your luggage, deduct the amount that the airline paid for necessary articles and file for the amount of the rest of your belongings plus the cost of your luggage.

When luggage is damaged, some airlines will request that you have your luggage repaired and they will reimburse you, while others will send it to their own repair shop. If you can't have your luggage repaired, negotiate for replacement costs.

Although having a wheelchair damaged during flight is unusual, it does happen. Don't panic. Since airline personnel often transport you in your wheelchair, they are likely to be present when the damage is discovered. If they aren't, get someone to report the incident and bring airline personnel to you. Often they will try to repair the chair right away or see that it is done as soon as possible. Carrying tools designed for your wheelchair is wise because mechanics can often get it working again.

My chair was dropped out of the airplane during unloading

in the Cairo, Egypt airport. I first showed my baggage claim to prove my case. Since this airport doesn't have wheelchairs, it was difficult to get to a taxi. Some people traveling on my tour assisted me to the hotel where the desk clerk called a rental agency and ordered a wheelchair for the rest of my stay. Make sure you save receipts of wheelchair rentals for presentation when you make claims for damage. This trip was the only time I didn't have a companion and I was determined never to travel alone again.

A wise precaution before leaving home is to take a picture of your wheelchair and write the model and serial numbers on a piece of paper for identification and proof of the condition of the wheelchair before you left home. This will assist you in your claims of damage or theft.

***Health Problems.*** If you become ill or involved in an accident, see Staying Healthy While Traveling, p. 47 , for advice on receiving medical care.

Although most medical insurance covers hospitals and doctors, ambulance service is usually not covered. Many special services required in an emergency are not covered and can cost thousands of dollars. You may buy additional insurance to cover these unexpected costs while traveling. Different companies offer different coverages. Compare benefits carefully to see if insurance will pay for emergency transportation more than once, if there are mileage and expense limits, and if coverage is applicable worldwide. Policies may be purchased from the following companies:[1]

International SOS Assistance, Inc./ P.O. Box 11568/ Philadelphia, Pennsylvania 19116, 215-244-1500 or/ outside of Philadelphia, 800-523-8930.
Fees are based on a daily, monthly or annual basis.

Near, Inc./ 1900 North MacArthur Boulevard, Suite 210/ Oklahoma City, Oklahoma 73127, 405-949-2500 or/ outside of Oklahoma State, 800-654-6700. Fees are daily or annual and can include other special coverage.

---

1. Paul Grimes, *Practical Traveler: If Illness Strikes One Far From Home*, New York Times, New York, New York.

MedHelp Overseas/ c/o International Underwriters/ Brokers, Inc./ 923 Investment Building, 1511 K Street, N.W./ Washington, D.C. 20005, 202-393-5500 or/ outside Washington, D.C., 800-336-3310. Fees are based on a daily rate with a minimum coverage.

There are many travel options offered with most comprehensive travel protection policies. Travel Insurance, PAC, Travelers Insurance Company, is a good policy. Ask your travel agent what coverage they offer. Some policies provide assistance besides just reimbursement for expenses. Such assistance includes advice in situations where you would welcome a knowledgeable person as you face a health emergency.

***Hotel Problems.*** It is not uncommon to have problems with hotels. Don't take a chance on unconfirmed reservations. Get confirmations in writing before you leave home. If you have not received an answer, send a telegram or overnight mail letter that insists the receiver sign a statement. Enclose a self-addressed, return envelope for your protection. Make sure to send deposits on rooms in a timely manner or you may not find a room available when you arrive. Deposit receipts or copies of checks plus written confirmation prove that you or your agent made the reservations. If rooms are inaccessible, inferior or unavailable, there will be no question as to your original requirements when you show your documentation.

It is more difficult to deal with hotel problems in foreign nations than at home because you are without Better Business Bureaus or Convention Bureaus to assist you. Also, when you are in a foreign country for a short period of time, it is impractical to threaten or actually sue for injustices. Naturally, foreign hotel personnel are well aware of your plight and use it to their advantage.

The best way to have your problems taken care of is to persuade hotel managers that they must accommodate your needs. If you have booked through a travel agent or with a tour, they will often help you since hotels are dependent on repeat trade from travel agents. Once, when I arrived to find my hotel filled and was sent to another hotel not nearly as nice or accessible, my travel agent negotiated a free stay at a hotel in the original chain the next time I traveled.

Hotels often overbook rooms just as airlines overbook flights. Ideally, hotels should provide equivalent accommodations. Unfortunately, sometimes a hotel will do nothing for you regardless of a commitment. Being nice and persuasive is your best weapon against hotel problems. However, if they are nasty, return righteous indignation for rudeness.

You have an obligation to the hotel to honor your confirmed reservation. You are under obligation to cancel by a stipulated date or you are responsible for paying for your room. Although hotels are supposed to try and rent the room to someone else, this doesn't always occur and you are liable for the expense. Just as it is difficult for you to sue in a foreign country, it is equally hard for them to take the same action against you. So, when you cancel, they usually take your advance deposit and are grateful for whatever they collected.

Hotels are only liable for personal injuries if they are negligent. It is difficult to collect if you fall down the stairs. Exceptions are sometimes made if you become ill resulting from the hotel's food or drink. Beware that if you are displeased with a hotel's service or policy and refuse to pay the bill, in most countries hotels are allowed to place a lien on your luggage and all possessions except the clothes you are wearing.

Sometimes American consulates are helpful in hotel or merchandise disputes. But since consulates are often under-staffed, they are more likely to assist you if your problem is with foreign government employees such as customs officials.

**Thefts.** Thiefs and pickpockets prevail both in the United States and abroad. Precautions will help prevent you from becoming a victim. The American Consulate in Rome advises travelers that hotel safes are the best places to store extra cash, travelers checks, credit cards, Eurail passes, airline tickets and jewelry. They also feel that shoulderbag pocketbooks should be carried on the side farthest from the street to discourage thefts by bikers or motorcyclists. For additional safety you should hold such bags just above the clasp and other types of pocketbooks close to your body. Pockets are a better place to carry passports than pocketbooks or wallets, and driver's licenses, identification, social security cards, pictures, letters and anything you value are safer in your hotel than with you when you are shopping, sightseeing or dining. Some other good tips are:

- Baggage should never be left unattended. Even locked suitcases can be broken into, so store valuables in the hotel safe.
- Leave nothing in parked cars.
- If parked cars must hold luggage, when eating in a restaurant, try and sit with a view of the car.
- Whenever possible, park cars in a public parking lot or garage.
- When hiring a native to watch your car; promise an extra tip if when you return nothing is stolen or has happened to the car.
- Don't put cameras or handbags on the floor, empty chairs, or the back of a chair.
- Hide your camera in your room, or, better yet, put it in the hotel safe when you aren't using it.
- Don't be careless or absentminded no matter how wonderful the sight you are observing.
- The less prosperous you look, the better off you are.
- Be more cautious in countries with a low standard of living.
- Beware of pickpockets at crowded tourist attractions, beaches, parks, zoos, and busy stores or marketplaces.
- Avoid unfamiliar streets after dark.
- Stay on well traveled highways.
- Don't leave valuables lying around your hotel room. They are tempting for theft, can be mislaid or swept into or under a bed or dresser.

Hotel thefts occur despite cautionary measures. In some countries, hotels are liable for destruction, loss or theft, even if they aren't responsible, while others will only do something if you can prove they were negligent. Hotels may limit their responsibility if you neglect to lock your doors or if signs or other notices requiring that valuables be placed in a safe exempt them from responsibility for the loss. Boarding houses may not be held to the same standards of liability as hotels, so be more careful of your possessions there.

Report all thefts as soon as possible. If robbery occurs in your hotel, tell the manager immediately. Make sure the local police are alerted. Put your losses in writing and leave a copy with the hotel manager and the police. If you become a victim outside the hotel, go to the nearest police station as soon as possible. Explain to the authorities the circumstances of the theft to the best of your abilities.

It's smart to insure your baggage and personal possessions before leaving home. Check your homeowners policy to see if it covers your valuables while traveling. If it doesn't, buy coverage.

If your passport is stolen, report it immediately to the police, embassy or local consulate. It is possible to replace your passport when you are in another country but it is time consuming and may delay your trip several days. You may not be able to cash travelers checks and will have other inconveniences while you are without proof of your identity.

Lost travelers checks are refundable if you have a record of the serial number of each check. That is why it is advisable to keep a copy of this list in a place separate from your checks. Notify the issuing bank by telephone and telegram. American Express will help you at most major airports. The reason for using tavelers checks is that your money will be refunded if lost or stolen.

If you lose a driver's license, report it to the police. It is useful to carry a copy of your license in case of emergencies.

If you lose your airline ticket, you must file a lost ticket refund form with the airline. It usually takes a few months for a refund so be prepared to spend money for your trip home.

***Out of Money.*** If you run out of money, don't despair. Go to a bank and request that funds be transferred from home. The local consulate will tell you which American banks have affiliates abroad who will perform this service. Be prepared and check with your bank before you leave home to get a list of affiliates.

Major credit cards are another source of funds. If you go to any bank that distributes your card, such as MasterCard or Visa, they will give you money up to your cash advance limit.

Family or friends can call Western Union to have money forwarded to you. Your rescuers need not leave home since Western Union will charge it to a credit card.

*If You Are Arrested.* [2]  Law enforcement systems outside the United States are stricter in some countries and more lenient in others. In most cases, tourists can resolve problems concerning the law without being arrested or jailed. Foreign countries are usually much stricter than the United States concerning the possession of controlled substances, and jail sentences of varying lengths are quite common. In some countries, people are thrown into terrible prisons for years for having a small amount of marijuana on them. Don't take a chance; take only those drugs prescribed by your doctor.

Under international law, tourists are subject to the same laws, rights and penalties as that country's citizens. United States citizens are not protected by the United States Constitution. Tourists must conform to a country's laws and penalties but aren't to be treated worse because they are visitors from another country. The most difficult problem facing tourists who are arrested in another country is not only ignorance of their rights but also often not knowing enough of the foreign language to understand what is happening to them. In many countries, you may have an interpreter, but finding one is not always possible.

Except for a few African countries, all nations are obligated by Article 36 of the Vienna Consular Convention to notify the nearest American consulate as soon as you are arrested or taken into custody. Different countries interpret their legal obligations differently. Some law enforcement officials are vague on "notification without delay" to the nearest American consulate. Some countries may hold someone for "investigation and questioning" for a week and then make a formal arrest. Notification isn't made until after the arrest.

When the American consul does arrive you will be told the

---

2. *Super Traveler*, Saul Millery, Holt, Rinehart and Winston, New York 1980.

legal procedures and your rights, and given a list of attorneys. The consul will make sure you haven't been mistreated because you are a U.S. citizen. If you have been mistreated, all the consul can do is file an official protest. If you are detained for a long time, the consulate will visit you about once a month to check on your treatment.

The consulate will notify the State Department of your arrest and will contact friends or relatives and relay any requests. Ask the consulate for an information packet on arrest and court procedures. What will happen to you will depend on where you were arrested and on what charges.

It pays to be cautious when traveling in another country. Be extra careful when traveling in rural areas of less sophisticated countries. Sometimes small village officials are not knowledge-able about legal rights and tend to ignore them. American consulates are far away and may not be reachable by phone. Don't let a good time make you forget all the safety measures that you know and use when in potentially dangerous situations at home.

**Uncomfortable Political Situations.** You may knowingly or innocently travel in an area with an unstable political climate. Know the possibilities that something negative might happen. Bombs or fighting can be a reality when traveling to Northern Ireland or Israel, but thousands of people think the benefits outweigh the potential liabilities and visit these two popular countries each year. I visited London during a series of bomb scares. However, there are many countries I would prefer not to visit because of political uncertainties. This is a personal deci-sion that each of us must make. Gather as much information as you can from your travel agent, newspapers and magazines and then make an intelligent decision.

Don't let this section frighten you into staying home. It is practical advice in case an emergency occurs. It will help you avoid disasters if possible, or at least let you know how to deal with unpleasant experiences that can happen to any traveler, not just the disabled.

# WHAT TRAVELING HAS DONE FOR ME

Before I became ill, I dreamed of visiting many different places around the world, but it wasn't until after I was disabled that I actually started to travel. When I was first forced to use a walker, I took a bus trip alone to New York City to prove to myself that I was not a prisoner of my disability. The freedom I lost was traded for an expanded view of the world. This impetus to travel soon became addictive. I have been to many places and there are many more I plan to see. I may have to postpone my trip to the Far East until that part of the world becomes more accessible, but I'm going.

Traveling has proven to be an enjoyable challenge. To me, it has meant that if I can travel, I can do anything. My sense of self-worth and independence have grown as I have met new and different challenges. Traveling has allowed me to fulfill my curiosity about many different places and people while giving me pleasure and excitement. Travel has also been a well needed respite from everyday struggles and problems. I have chosen to make traveling a priority in my life. My disability has not meant immobility. For we disabled can be "Traveling . . . Like Everybody Else."

# APPENDIX

## ACCESS INFORMATION IN THE UNITED STATES*

### UNITED STATES in general

*Airport Guide for the Handicapped and Elderly:* CHICAGO O'HARE INTERNATIONAL AIRPORT, Chicago Department of Aviation, City Hall, Room 1111, Chicago, Illinois 60602.

*Facilities and Services for the Handicapped:* NEWARK INTERNATIONAL, LA GUARDIA, AND KENNEDY INTERNATIONAL AIRPORTS, Port Authority of New York and New Jersey, Aviation Public Service Division, 1 World Trade Center, Room 65N, New York, New York 10048.

*Guide for the Handicapped:* DALLAS-FORT WORTH AIRPORT, Easter Seal Society for Crippled Children and Adults of Texas, Inc., 4429 N. Central Expressway, Dallas, Texas 75205.

*Guide for the Handicapped and Elderly:* LOS ANGELES INTERNATIONAL AIRPORT, Public Relations Bureau, Los Angeles Department of Airports, 1 World Way, Los Angeles, California 90009.

*Access National Parks:* A GUIDE FOR HANDICAPPED VISITORS (stock number 024–005–00691–5), by the National Park Service, Department of the Interior and available from Superintendent of Documents, U.S. Government Printing Office, Washington, D.C. 20402.

*Access to Corps of Engineers Lakes in Southeastern States* (A guide for handicapped visitors to Corps of Engineers Lakes in Alabama, Florida, Georgia, North Carolina, South Carolina and Virginia), U.S. Army Corps of Engineers, South Atlantic Division, Recreation Resource Management Branch, 510 Title Building, 30 Pryor Street S.W., Atlanta, Georgia 30303.

---

* International Directory of Access Guides, Travel Survey Department, Rehabilitation International USA, 20 West 40th Street, New York, NY 10018.

***Highway Rest Areas for Handicapped Travelers,*** President's Committee on Employment of the Handicapped, Washington, D.C. 20210.

***National Park Guide for the Handicapped*** (stock number 2405–0286), by the National Park Service, Department of the Interior and available from Superintendent of Documents, U.S. Government Printing Office, Washington, D.C. 20402.

### ALABAMA

BIRMINGHAM

***Birmingham, Alabama—***A GUIDE FOR THE AGED AND HANDI-CAPPED, The Mayor's Council for the Betterment of the Handicapped, 305 City Hall, 710 North 20th Street, Birmingham, Alabama 35203.

MONTGOMERY

***Access to Montgomery:*** A GUIDE FOR THE HANDICAPPED, by the Good Morning Kiwanis Club of Montgomery and available from Alabama Governor's Committee on Employment of the Handicapped, Box 11586, 2129 E. South Boulevard, Montgomery, Alabama 36198.

### ALASKA

ANCHORAGE

***The Anchorage Guide for the Physically Handicapped,*** by the Alaska Rehabilitation Association and available from Alaska Division of Vocational Rehabilitation, 4100 Spenard Road, Anchorage, Alaska 99503.

### ARKANSAS

HOT SPRINGS

***A Guide to Hot Springs for the Handicapped,*** The Garland County Easter Seal Society for Crippled Children and Adults, Inc., 2801 Lee Avenue, Little Rock, Arkansas 72205.

### CALIFORNIA

BEVERLY HILLS

***Around the Town with Ease—***A GUIDE FOR THE PHYSICALLY LIMITED PERSON, Junior League of Los Angeles, Beverly Wilshire Hotel, 9500 Wilshire Boulevard at Rodeo Drive, Beverly Hills, California 90212.

### EUREKA

***Access to Eureka for the Handicapped,*** by the Architectural Barriers Committee and available from Easter Seal Society for Crippled Children and Adults of Humboldt County, Box 996, 3289 Edgewood Drive, Eureka, California 95501.

### LOS ANGELES

***All About LAX,*** Los Angeles Department of Airports, 1 World Way, Los Angeles, California 90009.

***Los Angeles, Around the Town with Ease,*** Junior League of Los Angeles, Farmer's Market, Third and Fairfax, Los Angeles, California 90036.

***Guide for the Handicapped and Elderly:*** LOS ANGELES INTERNATIONAL AIRPORT, Public Relations Bureau, Los Angeles Department of Airports, 1 World Way, Los Angeles, California 90009.

### OAKLAND

***A Guide to Oakland and Parts of Berkeley for the Physically Disabled and Aging,*** Access California, Room 614, City Hall, Oakland, California 94612.

### PALO ALTO

***Getting Around in Palo Alto,*** City of Palo Alto, Department of Social and Community Services, 250 Hamilton Avenue, Palo Alto, California 94301.

### SACRAMENTO

***A Guidebook to Sacramento for the Physically Handicapped and Aging,*** California Association for the Physically Handicapped, P.O. Box 2252, Sacramento, California 95822.

### SAN DIEGO

***Freeways:*** SAN DIEGO DIRECTORY FOR THE DISABLED COMMUNITY, Able-Disabled Advocacy, Inc., 861 Sixth Avenue, Suite 610, San Diego, California 92101.

### SAN FRANCISCO

***Guide to San Francisco for the Handicapped,*** Easter Seal Society for Crippled Children and Adults of San Francisco, Inc., 1600 Lake Street, San Francisco, California 94121.

SANTA BARBARA

***Open Doors for the Handicapped in Santa Barbara,*** Easter Seal Society for Crippled Children and Adults of Santa Barbara County, 31 E. Canon Perdido, Santa Barbara, California 93101.

## CONNECTICUT

BRIDGEPORT/FAIRFIELD COUNTY

***Public Service Access Guide for Fairfield County,*** Ruth C. Gregory, EACH, 1830 Nicholas Avenue, Stratford, Connecticut 06497 *or* UCP Center, 130 Hunting Street, Bridgeport, Connecticut 06606.

HARTFORD

***An Access Guide for Greater Hartford,*** Architecture for Everyone Committee, Greater Hartford Chamber of Commerce, 250 Constitution Plaza, Hartford, Connecticut 06103.

NEW BRITAIN

***Your Key to New Britain:*** A HANDBOOK FOR THE HANDICAPPED, by the Junior League of New Britain and available from New Britain Chamber of Commerce, 127 Main Street, New Britain, Connecticut 06051 *or* The Society for Crippled Children and Adults, 682 Prospect Street, Hartford, Connecticut 06103.

NEW HAVEN

***Access New Haven,*** New Haven Office of Handicapped Services, 270 Orange Street, New Haven, Connecticut 06510 *or* RESPOND, Inc., 956 Chapel Street, New Haven, Connecticut 06510.

***A Register of Architecturally Surveyed Facilities in the New Haven Area,*** Woodbridge Rotary Club, c/o MITE Corp., 446 Blake Street, Woodbridge, Connecticut 06515.

STAMFORD

***The Directory,*** Easter Seal Rehabilitation Center of Southwestern Connecticut, 16 Palmer's Hill Road, Stamford, Connecticut 06902.

***A Guide to Southern Fairfield County for the Handicapped,*** Easter Seal Rehabilitation Center of Southwestern Connecticut, 150 Middlesex Road, Darien, Connecticut 06820.

***Southern Fairfield County Committee on Architecture for Everyone,*** 26 Palmer's Hill Road, Stamford, Connecticut 06902.

*Access Waterbury,* Easter Seal Rehabilitation Center of Greater Waterbury, 22 Tompkins Street, Waterbury, Connecticut 06708.

## DELAWARE

REHOBOTH BEACH

*Welcome Handicapped Visitors,* Rehoboth Beach Chamber of Commerce, 73 Rehoboth Avenue, Rehoboth, Delaware 19971 *or* Jo Anne Holson, Delmarva Easter Seal Rehabilitation Center, 204 E. North Street, Georgetown, Delaware 19947.

WILMINGTON/NORTHERN DELAWARE

*A Guide to Northern Delaware for the Disabled,* Easter Seal Society of Del-Mar, 2705 Baynard Boulevard, Wilmington, Delaware 19802.

*A Guide to Wilmington for the Handicapped,* Delaware Society for Crippled Children and Adults, Inc., 2705 Baynard Boulevard, Wilmington, Delaware 19802.

## DISTRICT OF COLUMBIA

*Access Washington:* A GUIDE TO METROPOLITAN WASHINGTON FOR THE PHYSICALLY DISABLED, Information Center for Handicapped Individuals, Inc., 120 C Street, N.W., Washington, D.C. 20001.

*The Deaf Person's Quick Guide to Washington (D.C.),* Alice Hagemeyer, c/o Martin Luther King Memorial Library, 901 G Street, N.W., Room 410, Washington, D.C. 20001.

*Washington, D.C.:* A GUIDE TO WASHINGTON FOR THE PHYSICALLY HANDICAPPED, The D.C. Society for Crippled Children, 2800 13th Street, N.W., Washington, D.C. 20009 *or* The Maryland Society for Crippled Children and Adults, 9422 Annapolis Road, Lanham, Maryland 20801 *or* The Northern Virginia Society for Crippled Children and Adults, 3501 Columbia Pike, Arlington, Virginia 22204.

## FLORIDA

DAYTONA BEACH

*Guide to Daytona Beach Area,* The Palmetto Club Juniors of Daytona Beach, Florida, Palmetto Women's Club, 1000 S. Beach, Daytona Beach, Florida 32014.

*Access to Gainsville,* by the Department of Rehabilitative Services of Alachua County and available from Gainsville Chamber of Commerce, 300 E. University, Gainsville, Florida 32602.

*Guide for the Handicapped:* JACKSONVILLE, by the Jacksonville Junior Services League and available from Society for Crippled Children and Adults of Northeastern Florida, 1056 Oak Street, Jacksonville, Florida 32204.

*Accessibility Guide to South Brevard,* Easter Seal Rehabilitation Center, 450 E. Sheridan Road, Melbourne, Florida 32901.

*Access Miami:* A GUIDE FOR THE HANDICAPPED, City of Miami, Department of Leisure Services, Programs for the Handicapped, 2600 S. Bayshore Drive, Box 330708, Miami, Florida 33133.

*Wheelchair Directory of Greater Miami,* Florida Paraplegic Association, Inc., ATTN: Sal Zitter, 1366 13th Terrace, Miami Beach, Florida 33139 *or* City of Miami, Department of Leisure Services, 2600 S. Bayshore Drive, Box 330708, Miami, Florida 33133.

*Orlando's Guide for the Handicapped,* by the Orlando Area Tourist Trade Association and available from Chamber of Commerce, Box 1234, Orlando, Florida 32802 *or* Florida Easter Seal Society, 231 E. Colonial Drive, Orlando, Florida 32801.

*Guide to Orlando-Winter Park* GUIDEBOOK FOR THE PHYSICALLY HANDICAPPED, DISABLED VETERANS, SENIOR CITIZENS, The Florida Society for Crippled Children and Adults, Inc., 231 E. Colonial Drive, Orlando, Florida 32801.

*Accessibility:* LOWER PINELLAS COUNTY, Easter Seal Rehabilitation Center, 7671 Highway 19, Pinellas Park, Florida 33565 *or* City of St. Petersburg, Box 2842, St. Petersburg, Florida 33731.

*Guide to Sarasota for the Handicapped,* Happiness House Rehabilitation Center, Inc., 401 Braden Avenue, Sarasota, Florida 33580.

*Guide to the Tampa Area for the Physically Handicapped,* by Hillsborough Community College and available from Easter Seal Society for Crippled Children and Adults of Hillsborough County, A. Pickens Cole Easter Seal Center, 2401 E. Henry Avenue, Tampa, Florida 33610.

## GEORGIA

ATLANTA

*A Guidebook to Atlanta for the Handicapped,* Georgia Easter Seal Society, 3254 Northside Parkway, N.W. Atlanta, Georgia 30327 *or* Georgia Society for Crippled Children and Adults, Inc., 30 Pryor Street S.W., Atlanta, Georgia 30303.

*Getting About Atlanta*—GUIDE FOR THE PHYSICALLY HANDICAPPED AND AGED, Georgia Society for Crippled Children and Adults, 1211 Spring Street N.W., Atlanta, Georgia 30309.

ALBANY

*Guide for the Handicapped to the Greater Albany Area,* The Southwest Georgia Area Easter Seal Rehabilitation Center, 1906 Palmyra Road, Albany, Georgia 31701.

## HAWAII

*Hawaii Visitors Bureau Member Hotel Guide* (access indicated), Hawaii Visitors Bureau, Suite 801, 2270 Kalakaua Avenue, Honolulu, Hawaii 96815.

HONOLULU

*Aloha Guide to Oahu for the Handicapped,* Hawaii Society for Crippled Children and Adults, 335 Merchant Street, Room 215, Honolulu, Hawaii 96822.

*A Pictorial Aloha Guide to Honolulu for Handicapped Travelers,* Hawaii Visitors Bureau, Suite 801, 2270 Kalakaua Avenue, Honolulu, Hawaii 96815.

***Guide for the Handicapped to Maui, Hawaii,*** by the Maui Jaycees and the Easter Seal Society of Maui County and available from Easter Seal Society of Maui County, 95 Mahalani Street, Wailuku, Hawaii 96793.

***Maui Easter Seal Society***—GUIDE FOR THE HANDICAPPED, Maui Units, National Easter Seal Society for Crippled Children and Adults, Inc., P.O. Box 183, Kahukui, Hawaii 96732.

## ILLINOIS

***Handicapped Individual's Guide to Illinois Recreation Areas,*** Dr. Silas P. Singh, Ph.D., Handicapped Program Coordinator, Department of Conservation, 405 E. Washington, Springfield, Illinois 62701.

BLOOMINGTON-NORMAL

***A Guide to Bloomington-Normal for the Handicapped,*** Mayor's Committee on Employment of the Handicapped, c/o City Hall, Bloomington, Illinois 61701.

CARBONDALE

***Carbondale Guide for the Handicapped,*** Easter Seal Society of Southern Illinois, Box 3249, Carbondale, Illinois 62901.

CHICAGO

***A Guide to the Chicago Loop for the Handicapped,*** The Chicago Easter Seal Society, 116 S. Michigan Avenue, Chicago, Illinois 60603.

***Access Chicago:*** A GUIDE TO THE CITY, Research Dissemination Rehabilitation Institute of Chicago, 345 E. Superior Street, Chicago, Illinois 60611.

SPRINGFIELD

***Building Access Guide for the Handicapped and Aging,*** Eileen McCune, Chairperson, Altrusa Club of Springfield, 623 East Adams Street, Springfield, Illinois 62706.

## INDIANA

BLOOMINGTON

***Moving Ahead***—MOBILITY BARRIERS OVERCOME IN BLOOMINGTON, INDIANA, Social Services, Bloomington Hospital, 605 West Second Street, Bloomington, Indiana 47401.

EVANSVILLE

**A Guide for the Handicapped for Evansville,** by the Junior League of Evansville, Indiana and available from Vanderburgh County Society for Crippled Children, 3701 Bellemeade Avenue, Evansville, Indiana 47715.

INDIANAPOLIS

**Navigation Unlimited in Indianapolis,** Marion County Muscular Dystrophy Foundation, 616 N. Alabama Street, Room 214, Indianapolis, Indiana 46204.

## IOWA

CEDAR RAPIDS

**Cedar Rapids Area Accessibility Guide,** Kirkwood Community College, Skill Center Division, Box 2068, Cedar Rapids, Iowa 52406

DES MOINES

**A Guidebook to Des Moines for the Handicapped,** Alpha Omicron Alpha Chapter, Alpha Chi Omega, Des Moines, Iowa.

DUBUQUE

**A Guidebook to Accessible Places in Dubuque,** Project Access Dubuque, Box 361, Dubuque, Iowa 52001.

## KANSAS

TOPEKA

**Facilities Directory:** A GUIDE TO ACCESSIBLE ESTABLISHMENTS, by the Topeka-Shawnee City Human Relations Commission and available from Division for the Disabled, City of Topeka, City Hall, Room 54, Topeka, Kansas 66603.

**Facilities Directory:** A GUIDE TO BARRIER FREE ESTABLISHMENTS 1974-75, Division for the Disabled, City of Topeka, City Hall, Room 54, Topeka, Kansas 66603.

WICHITA

**A Guide for the Disabled of Wichita,** by the Kansas Easter Seal Society, Kansas Paralysis Chapter, and Wichita Volunteers and available from Easter Seal Society for Crippled Children and Adults of Kansas, 3701 Plaza Drive, Topeka, Kansas 66609.

# KENTUCKY

ASHLAND

*A Guide to Ashland for the Handicapped,* Kentucky Society for Crippled Children, 233 East Broadway, Louisville, Kentucky 40202.

LOUISVILLE

*A Guide to Louisville for the Handicapped,* Kentucky Society for Crippled Children, Inc., 233 East Broadway, Louisville, Kentucky 40202.

MURRAY/AURORA

*Access Guide:* RESTAURANT FACILITIES, Rehabilitation Education Program, Department of Professional Studies, Murray State University, Murray, Kentucky 42071 *or* Murray-Calloway County Chamber of Commerce, 300 Maple, Murray, Kentucky 42071.

# LOUISIANA

BATON ROUGE

*Baton Rouge*—A GUIDE FOR THE HANDICAPPED, the Junior League of Baton Rouge, Baton Rouge, Louisiana *or* Easter Seal Society for Crippled Children and Adults of Louisiana, Inc., 200 Henry Clay Avenue, New Orleans, Louisiana 70118.

NEW ORLEANS

*Access New Orleans,* Easter Seal Society for Crippled Childrenand Adults of Louisiana, Inc., Box 8425, Metairie, Louisiana 70011.

*Rolling Tour of the French Quarter,* Easter Seal Society for Crippled Children and Adults of Louisiana, Inc. Box 8425, Metairie, Louisiana 70011.

*A Guide to New Orleans for the Handicapped,* The Louisiana Chapter, National Society for Crippled Children and Adults, Inc., 843 Carondelet Street, New Orleans, Louisiana 70130.

SHREVEPORT

*A Guide to Facilities in Shreveport and Bossier City,* Community Council Office, 1702 Irving Place, Shreveport, Louisiana 71101.

## MAINE

*Easy Wheelin,* City of Portland Parks and Recreation Leisure Center, YMCA Building, 70 Forest Avenue, Portland, Maine 04101

## MARYLAND

BALTIMORE

*Ready/Set/Go!* BALTIMORE GUIDEBOOK FOR THE PHYSICALLY DISABLED, by Rhoda Eskwith and Ellen Christiansen and available from the League for the Handicapped, 1111 East Cold Spring Lane, Baltimore, Maryland 21239.

## MASSACHUSETTS

BOSTON

*Wheeling Through Boston,* Easter Seal Society, 14 Somerset Street, Boston, Massachusetts 02108.

*At Your Service,* Massachusetts Rehabilitation Hospital, c/o Recreation Therapy Department, 125 Nashua Street, Boston, Massachusetts 02114.

CAMBRIDGE

*Access to Cambridge* Alpha Chi Chapter, Alpha Phi Omega National Service Fraternity, Massachusetts Institute of Technology, Cambridge, Massachusetts 02139 *or* Easter Seal Society, 14 Somerset Street, Boston, Massachusetts 02108.

FALL RIVER

*The Greater Fall River Area Handbook for the Handicapped,* Fall River Chamber of Commerce, 101 Rock Street, Fall River, Massachusetts 02721.

GREENFIELD

*A Guide to Greenfield for the Physically Disabled and Aging,* Easter Seal Society for Crippled Children and Adults of Massachusetts, Inc., 30 Highland Street, Worcester, Massachusetts 01608.

SPRINGFIELD

*A Guide to Springfield for the Physically Handicapped and Aging,* Easter Seal Society for Crippled Children and Adults of

Massachusetts, Inc., 380 Union Street, West Springfield, Massachusetts 01089 *or* 145 Spring Street, Springfield, Massachusetts 01103 *or* 9 Newbury Street, Boston, Massachusetts 02116.

WORCESTER

*A Guide to Worcester for the Physically Handicapped and Aging,* Easter Seal Society for Crippled Children and Adults of Massachusetts, 37 Harvard Street, Worcester, Massachusetts 01608.

## MICHIGAN

*Travel Michigan:* HANDICAPPERS MINI-GUIDE, Travel Bureau, Michigan Department of Commerce, Box 30226, Lansing, Michigan 48909.

DETROIT

*Guide to Detroit for the Handicapped,* by the Tau Beta Association and available from Rehabilitation Institute, 261 Mack Boulevard, Detroit, Michigan 48201.

*Guide to Detroit for the Handicapped,* Tau Beta Association, 51 West Warren Avenue, Detroit, Michigan 48201.

FLINT

*A Guide for the Handicapped,* Easter Seal Society of Genessee County, 1420 W. Third Avenue, Flint, Michigan 48504.

GRAND RAPIDS

*A Guide to Grand Rapids for the Handicapped,* Kent County Society for Crippled Children and Adults, Inc., 218 Hollister Avenue S.E., Grand Rapids, Michigan 49506.

LANSING

*Access Lansing,* The Center for Handicapped Affairs, 1026 E. Michigan Avenue, Lansing, Michigan 48912.

*A Guide for the Handicapped to the Greater Lansing Area,* Ingham Country Society for Crippled Children and Adults, 113 Lapeer Street, Lansing, Michigan 48933.

## MINNESOTA

*Easy Wheelin' in Minnesota,* Robert R. Peters, 1 Timberglade Road, Bloomington, Minnesota 55437.

*A Guidebook to Duluth for the Handicapped,* Nat G. Polinsky Rehabilitation Center, 530 East Second Street, Duluth, Minnesota 55805.

*Access Rochester,* Hiawatha Valley Chapter, National Spinal Cord Injury Foundation, Box 136, Rochester, Minnesota 55901.

## MISSISSIPPI

JACKSON

*A Key to Jackson for the Physically Limited,* by the Junior League of Jackson and available from Mississippi Easter Seal Society, Box 4958, Jackson, Mississippi 39216.

*A Guidebook to Jackson for the Disabled,* Mississippi Easter Seal Society, 408 West Pascagoula Street, Jackson, Mississippi 39567.

## MISSOURI

COLUMBIA

*Access Columbia, MO.,* College of Home Economics, University of Missouri-Columbia, 329 Stanley Hall, Columbia, Missouri 65211.

KANSAS CITY

*Accessibility Directory:* KANSAS CITY, by the Architecture Barrier Committee and available from ACCESS, 3011 Baltimore, Kansas City, Missouri 64108.

ST. LOUIS

*St. Louis Has It A to Z for the Handicapped,* Easter Seal Society of Missouri-St. Louis Region, 4108 Lindell Boulevard, St. Louis, Missouri 63108.

## MONTANA

GREAT FALLS

*Guide to Great Falls for the Handicapped,* by the Community Concern Class of Charles M. Russell High School and available from Easter Seal Society for Crippled Children and Adults of Montana, State Headquarters, 4400 Central Avenue,

Great Falls, Montana 59401 *or* Great Falls Area Chamber of Commerce, Great Falls, Montana 59401.

## NEBRASKA

### LINCOLN

*A Guidebook to Lincoln for the Handicapped,* Larry Westphalen, Chairman, Mayor's Committee for Employment of the Physically Handicapped, 1120 Colony Lane, Lincoln, Nebraska 68505.

### OMAHA

*Accessible Building and Businesses in Omaha, Nebraska,* Easter Seal Society for Crippled Children and Adults, 12177 Pacific Street, Omaha, Nebraska 68154.

*A Guide to Omaha for the Handicapped,* Easter Seal Society for Crippled Children and Adults, WOW Building, Room 430, 1319 Farnam, Omaha, Nebraska 68102.

## NEVADA

### LAS VEGAS

*Access Las Vegas,* Governor's Committee on Employment of the Handicapped, State Mail Room, Las Vegas, Nevada 89158.

### RENO/SPARKS/CARSON CITY

*Access Reno, Sparks, Carson City:* A GUIDEBOOK FOR THE HANDICAPPED TRAVELER, Governor's Committee on Employment of the Handicapped, Kinkead Building, 5th floor, State Capital Complex, Carson City, Nevada 89710.

## NEW HAMPSHIRE

### THE HAMPTONS

*A Guide to the Hamptons,* Mrs. Sharon Parker, 548 Lafayette Road, Hampton, New Hampshire 03842.

## NEW JERSEY

### HACKENSACK

*A Guide to Hackensack for the Handicapped,* Easter Seal Society for Crippled Children and Adults of New Jersey, 171 Atlantic Street, Hackensack, New Jersey 07601.

### HIGHTSTOWN AND EAST WINDSOR

*Architectural Barrier Guide for the Handicapped,* Easter

Seal Society for Crippled Children and Adults, 300 Main Street, Orange, New Jersey 07050.

*A Guide for the Handicapped,* Easter Seal Society for Crippled Children and Adults, Inc., 300 Main Street, Orange, New Jersey 07050.

MONMOUTH COUNTY

*A Guide for the Handicapped,* Community Services Council for Monmouth County, Inc., One Third Avenue, Long Branch, New Jersey 07740.

SCOTCH PLAINS AND FANWOOD

*Scotch Plains and Fanwood for the Handicapped and Aging,* Easter Seal Society for Crippled Children and Adults, Inc., 300 Main Street, Orange, New Jersey 07050.

TEANECK

*A Guidebook to Teaneck for the Handicapped,* Easter Seal Society for Crippled Children and Adults of Bergen County, Inc., 799 Main Street, Hackensack, New Jersey 07601.

WARREN COUNTY

*Guide to Warren County, New Jersey,* Comeback, Inc., 16 W. 46th Street, New York, New York 10036.

WEST ESSEX

*Guidebook for the Handicapped—West Essex Area,* Easter Seal Society for Crippled Children and Adults of New Jersey, Inc., 799 Main Street, Hackensack, New Jersey 07601.

## NEW YORK

*I Love New York Travel Guide (access indicated),* includes coverage of Adirondacks, Catskills, Finger Lakes, Hudson Valley, Saratoga Region, Niagara Frontier, Thousand Islands, Long Island and available from New York State Department of Commerce, 99 Washington Avenue, Albany, New York 12210 *or* New York State Easter Seal Society, 194 Washington Avenue, Albany, New York 12210.

*New York State Thruway Facilities for Handicapped Travelers,* New York State Thruway Authority, 200 Southern Boulevard, Albany, New York 12201.

***Tips for the Physically Handicapped Accessibility Guide (a guide to cultural facilities),*** The Lincoln Center Public Information Department, 140 W. 65th Street, New York, New York 10023.

ALBANY/SCHENECTADY/TROY

***Access to Capitaland,*** by the Junior Leagues of Albany, Schenectady and Troy and available from Junior League of Schenectady, Box 857, Schenectady, New York 12301.

BUFFALO/LOCKPORT/NIAGARA FALLS

***Guide for the Disabled and Elderly,*** Tri-City Director, Building Barriers Committee, Rehabilitation Association of Western New York, P.O. Box 74, Buffalo, New York 14205.

HUNTINGTON

***Access Huntington:*** DIRECTORY OF ACCESSIBLE BUILDINGS, Town of Huntington, Services for the Handicapped, 423 Park Avenue, Huntington, New York 11743.

KINGSTON/ULSTER COUNTY

***Access Ulster County,*** Easter Seal Society, 855 Central Avenue, Albany, New York 12206.

NEW YORK CITY

***A Guide to New York City for Persons with Physical Limitations,*** The Easter Seal Society, 185 Madison Avenue, New York, New York 10016.

***Access New York,*** Institute of Rehabilitation Medicine, ATTN: Publications Office, New York University Medical Center, 400 E. 34th Street, New York, New York 10016.

***The Brooklyn Public Library:*** FACILITIES, SERVICES, ACCESSIBILITY, available with a stamped, self-addressed envelope from Brooklyn Public Library, ATTN: Public Relations, Grand Army Plaza, Brooklyn, New York 11238.

***Catholic Churches and All Parochial Facilities in Brooklyn and Queens Accessible to the Handicapped,*** Office for the Handicapped, Brooklyn Catholic Charities, 191 Joralemon Street, Brooklyn, New York 11201.

***I Love New York City,*** New York State Easter Seal Society, One Park Avenue, Suite 1815, New York, New York 10018.

*A Handicapped Person's Guide to Rochester,* Crippled Children's Society of Monroe County, Inc., 28 Euclid Street, Rochester, New York 14604.

*The People's Accessibility Guide to Greater Rochester, New York,* by Handicapped Independence H.E.R.E., Inc., and available from Easter Seal Society of Monroe County, Inc., 55 St. Paul Street, Rochester, New York 14604 *or* Handicapped Independence, 1400 Mount Hope Avenue, Rochester, New York 14620.

SYRACUSE

*See Syracuse*—A GUIDE FOR THE HANDICAPPED, Easter Seal Society, 1103 State Tower Building, Syracuse, New York 13202

UTICA

*Guide for the Physically Handicapped and Aged,* Mohawk Valley Easter Seal Society, 287 Genesee Street, Utica, New York 13501.

WESTCHESTER COUNTY

*A Guide to Lower Central Westchester County for the Handicapped,* Westchester Society for Crippled Children and Adults, Inc., 151 East Post Road, White Plains, New York 10601.

## NORTH CAROLINA

ASHEVILLE

*Guide to Asheville for the Disabled and Aging,* The Blue Ridge Regional Chapter, North Carolina Easter Seal Society, Asheville, North Carolina 28804.

CHARLOTTE

*Guide to Charlotte for the Handicapped,* Mecklenburg County Society for Crippled Children and Adults, Inc., 1420 East 7th Street, Charlotte, North Carolina 28204.

GREENSBORO

*A Guide for the Physically Handicapped,* by the Council on Conventions and Trade Shows, the City of Greensboro and the Easter Seal Society and available from Accessibility Task Force, Greensboro Chamber of Commerce, Box 3246, Greensboro, North Carolina 27402.

*Orange County Guide to Family Resources,* by the Orange County Commission for Women and the Orange County Mental Health Association and available from Orange County Commission for Women, 131 Court Street, Hillsborough, North Carolina 27278.

WINSTON-SALEM

*Twin-Cities Building Directory for the Handicapped,* Easter Seal Society, 1020 Brookstown Avenue, Winston-Salem, North Carolina 27101.

## NORTH DAKOTA

*North Dakota Highway System:* REST AREAS, North Dakota State Highway Department, Design Division, Bismark, North Dakota 58505.

JAMESTOWN

*A Guidebook for Jamestown for the Handicapped,* Easter Seal Society for Crippled Children and Adults of North Dakota, 422 Second Avenue Northwest, Jamestown, North Dakota 58401.

VALLEY CITY

*A Guidebook to Valley City for the Handicapped,* Easter Seal Society for Crippled Children and Adults of North Dakota, 422 Second Avenue Northwest, Jamestown, North Dakota 58401.

## OHIO

AKRON

*Akron Area Guide for the Handicapped,* The Junior League of Akron, Ohio, 929 West Market Street, Akron, Ohio 44313.

CANTON

*Guide to Canton for the Handicapped,* Goodwill Industries and Rehabilitation Clinic, 408 Ninth Southwest, Canton, Ohio 44703.

CINCINNATI

*Greater Cincinnati Guidebook for the Handicapped,* Public Health Federation, 2400 Reading Road, Cincinnati, Ohio 45202.

CLEVELAND

*A Guide to Cleveland for the Handicapped,* Vocational Guidance and Rehabilitation Services, Rehabilitation Center, 2239 East 55th Street, Cleveland, Ohio 44103 *or* Easter Seal Society, 20475 Farnsleigh Road, Shaker Heights, Ohio 44122 *or* National Council of Jewish Women, 3535 Lee Road, Shaker Heights, Ohio 44120.

COLUMBUS

*Columbus Guide for the Handicapped,* Goodwill Industries of Central Ohio, 1331 Edgehill Road, Columbus, Ohio 43215.

DAYTON

*A Guide to Dayton for the Handicapped,* The Junior League of Dayton, Ohio, Inc., Dayton, Ohio 45402 *or* Dayton Goodwill Industries, 201 West First Street, Dayton, Ohio 45402.

STEUBENVILLE

*A Guide to Steubenville, Ohio for the Handicapped,* Steubenville Area Chamber of Commerce, Steubenville, Ohio 43952.

TOLEDO

*A Guide to Toledo for the Handicapped,* Toledo Society for the Handicapped, 5605 Monroe Street, Sylvania, Ohio 43560.

## OKLAHOMA

TULSA

*A Guide to Tulsa for the Handicapped,* Mrs. Ralph L. Franklin, Altruistic Chairman, Tulsa Alumnae Chapter of Alpha Chi Omega, 2939 South Cincinnati, Tulsa, Oklahoma 74114.

## OREGON

OSWEGO LAKE

*A Guide for the Handicapped,* Oregon Society for Crippled Children and Adults, Inc., 5757 Macadam Avenue, Portland, Oregon 97201.

PORTLAND

*Circling the City,* Junior League of Portland, Oregon, 4838 S.W. Scholls Ferry Road, Portland, Oregon 97225 *or* Oregon Society for Crippled Children and Adults, Inc., 5757 Macadam Avenue, Portland, Oregon 97201.

***A Guide for the Handicapped Living in the Portland Area:*** INDIVIDUALS, AGENCIES, AND FACILITIES SERVING THE HANDICAPPED, Portland Community College, Handicapped Student Service Office, 12000 S.W. 49th Avenue, Portland, Oregon 97219.

### PENNSYLVANIA

BUCKS COUNTY

***Access Bucks County,*** Bucks County Easter Seal Center, 2400 Trenton Road, Levittown, Pennsylvania 19056.

DELAWARE COUNTY

***Guide to Delaware County for the Handicapped,*** Delaware County Easter Seal Rehabilitation Center, 468 N. Middletown Road, Media, Pennsylvania 19063.

ERIE

***Accessibility Guide,*** The Task Force, 645 East 23rd Street, Erie, Pennsylvania 16503.

PHILADELPHIA

***A Guide to Philadelphia for the Handicapped,*** Mayor's Office for the Handicapped, Room 427, City Hall Annex, Philadelphia, Pennsylvania 19107.

PITTSBURGH

***Access:*** A GUIDE TO THE CAMPUS OF THE UNIVERSITY OF PITTSBURGH, Access, Office of Special Student Services, 507 Schenley Hall, University of Pittsburgh, Pittsburgh, Pennsylvania 15260.

***A Guide to Pittsburgh for the Handicapped,*** OPEN DOORS FOR THE HANDICAPPED, 1013 Brintell Street, Pittsburgh, Pennsylvania 15201.

STATE COLLEGE

***A Guide to Downtown State College for the Disabled and Aging,*** Easter Seal Society for Crippled Children and Adults of Centre and Clinton Counties, 1300 S. Allen Street, State College, Pennsylvania 16801.

### RHODE ISLAND

***Guide to Rhode Island for the Handicapped,*** Crippled Children and Adults of Rhode Island, Inc., 333 Grotto Avenue, Providence, Rhode Island 02906.

## SOUTH CAROLINA

CHARLESTON

*Access Charleston,* Charleston County Park, Recreation and Tourism Commission, Box 834, Charleston, South Carolina 29402.

COLUMBIA

*Access Columbia,* by the Pilot Club of Columbia and available from Columbia Chamber of Commerce, 1308 Laurel Street, Columbia, South Carolina 29201.

## SOUTH DAKOTA

*Wheelchair Vacations in the Black Hills and Badlands of South Dakota,* by the State of South Dakota and available from Black Hills, Badlands and Lakes Association, Box 539, Sturgis, South Dakota 57785.

*Wheelchair Vacationing in South Dakota,* South Dakota Division of Tourism, Joe Foss Building, Pierre, South Dakota 57501 *or* Handicapped Citizens of South Dakota, Box 8005, Rapid City, South Dakota 57701.

## TENNESSEE

CHATTANOOGA

*The Disabled Visitor's Guide to the Chattanooge Area,* Chattanooga Area Convention and Visitors Bureau, Civic Forum, 1001 Market Street, Chattanooga, Tennessee 37402.

MEMPHIS

*A Guide to Memphis for the Handicapped,* MEMPHIS GUIDE FOR THE HANDICAPPED AND AGING, Easter Seal Society for Crippled Children and Adults of Shelby County, Inc., 1280 Farmville Road, Memphis, Tennessee 38121.

NASHVILLE

*A Guidebook to Nashville for the Handicapped and Aging,* Davidson County Committee, Easter Seal Society for Crippled Children and Adults of Tennessee, 424 Seventh Avenue, Nashville, Tennessee 37203.

# TEXAS

***Access Austin:*** A GUIDE TO AUSTIN FOR MOBILITY IMPAIRED PERSONS, MIGHT, Chapter II, Box 5746, Austin, Texas, 78763.

***Guide to the University of Texas at Austin for the Physically Handicapped,*** Services for Handicapped Students, Student Services Building, Room 2.116, P.O. Box 7849, University of Texas, Austin, Texas 78712.

DALLAS

***Access Dallas '77,*** by the Committee for the Removal of Architectural Barriers and available from Easter Seal Society, 4429 N. Central Expressway, Dallas, Texas 75205.

***A Guide to Dallas for the Handicapped,*** Texas Society for Crippled Children and Adults Inc., 4429 N. Central Expressway, Dallas, Texas 75205.

GONZALES

***Wheelin' Around Texas,*** Former Patient Association, Texas Rehabilitation Association, P.O. Box 58, Gonzalez, Texas 78625.

HOUSTON

***Guide to Houston for the Handicapped,*** Texas Institute of Rehabilitation and Research, 1333 Moursund Avenue, Houston, Texas 77030 *or* Coalition for Barrier-Free Living, Box 20803, Houston, Texas 77025.

MIDLAND

***Getting Around Midland,*** by the Junior League of Midland and available from Easter Seal Society, 4429 N. Central Expressway, Dallas, Texas 75205.

SAN ANTONIO

***Access San Antonio,*** Bexar County Easter Seal Society, 2203 Babcock Road, San Antonio, Texas 78229.

# UTAH

SALT LAKE CITY

***Access Salt Lake,*** Division of Rehabilitation Services, Utah State Board for Vocational Education, 250 E., 500 South Street, Salt Lake City, Utah 84111.

## VIRGINIA

NORFOLK/TIDEWATER REGION

***Tidewater Access Guide for the Handicapped,*** Norfolk Chamber of Commerce, Research Department, 420 Bank Street, Box 327, Norfolk, Virginia 23501.

***A Guide to Norfolk for the Handicapped and Aging,*** Health and Information Center, 100-A Royster Building, Norfolk, Virginia 23501.

RICHMOND

***Richmond Guide for the Handicapped and Aging,*** Easter Seal Society for Crippled Children and Adults, 3212 Cutshaw Avenue, Richmond, Virginia 23230.

ROANOKE VALLEY

***Guide for the Handicapped and Aging,*** Secretary, Mayor's Committee on Employment of the Handicapped, P.O. Box 61, Roanoke, Virginia 24002.

WILLIAMSBURG

***Guide for the Handicapped to Colonial Williamsburg,*** Colonial Williamsburg Foundation, Information Center, Colonial Williamsburg, Virginia 23185.

## WASHINGTON

SEATTLE

***Access Seattle,*** Easter Seal Society for Crippled Children and Adults, Attention: Barbara Allen, 521 Second Avenue West, Seattle, Washington 98119.

SPOKANE

***Guide to Spokane Area for the Handicapped,*** Easter Seal Society for Crippled Children and Adults of Washington, W. 510 Second Avenue, Spokane, Washington 99204.

## WEST VIRGINIA

***West Virginia Travel Guide for the Handicapped,*** WV Rehabilitation Association, Structural Barriers Program, 1427 Lee Street East, Charleston, West Virginia 25301.

*Wheeling Through Wheeling,* Wheeling-Ohio County Planning Commission, Room 305, City-County Building, 1600 Chapline Street, Wheeling, West Virginia 26003.

## WISCONSIN

MILWAUKEE

*A Guide to Milwaukee for the Handicapped,* The Easter Seal Society for Crippled Children and Adults of Milwaukee County, Inc., 5225 W. Burleigh Street, Milwaukee, Wisconsin 53210.

---

# AMERICAN FOREIGN SERVICE POSTS

**Argentina**
Buenos Aires, 4300 Colombia, 1425
Phone: 774-8811

**Australia**
Canberra, Moonah Place, Canberra
A.C.T. 2600, Phone: (062) 73-3711

**Austria**
Vienna, IX Boltzmangasse 16, A-1091
Phone: (222) 346611, 347511

Salzburg, 1 Franz Josefs, Kai, Room 302
Phone: 46461

**Bahamas**
Nassau, Mosmar Building, Queen Street
Phones: (809) 322-1700, 322-1811

**Belgium**
Brussels, 27 Boulevard de Regent
Phone: 513-3830

**Bermuda**
Hamilton, Vallis Building, Front Street
Phone: 295-1342

## Bolivia

La Paz, Banco Popular Del Peru Building
Corner of Calles Mercado y Colon,
Phone: 50251

## Brazil

Brasilia, Lote No. 3, Avenida das Nacoes
Phone: (0612) 223-0120

Rio de Janeiro, Avenida Presidente
Wilson, 147, Phones: (021) 252-8055
252-8056, 252-8057

## Canada

Ottawa, 100 Wellington Street, K1P 5T1
Phone: (613) 238-5335

Montreal, Suite 1122, South Tower, Place
Desjardins, P.O. Box 65, H5B 1G1
Phone: (514) 281-1886

Quebec, 1 Avenue Ste. Genevieve, G1R 4A7
Phone: (418) 692-2095

Toronto, 360 University Avenue
Phone: (416) 595-1700

## Chile

Santiago, Codina Building, 1343 Agustinas
Phones: 710133/90, 710326/75

## China, People's Republic of

Peking, Kuang Hua Lu
Phone: 522-033

## Colombia

Bogota, Calle 37, 8-40
Phone: 285-1300

## Denmark

Copenhagen, Dag Hammarskjold Ahe 24
Phone: 42-31-44

## Ecuador

Quito, 120 Avenida Patria
Phone: 548-000

**Egypt, Arab Republic of**

Cairo, 5 Sharia Latin America, P.O. Box 10

Phones: 28211, 28219

**Finland**

Helsinki, Itainen Puisotie 14A

Phone: 171931

**France**

Paris, 2 Avenue Gabriel

Phones: 296-1202, 261-8075

**German Democratic Republic**

Berlin, Neustaedtische Kirchstrasse 4-5, 108 Berlin

Phone: 2202741

**Germany, Federal Republic of**

Bonn, Deichmannsaue 5300

Phone: (02221) 89-55

Berlin, Clayallee 170, D-1000 Berlin 33 (Dahlem)

Phone: (030) 832-40-87

**Greece**

Athens, 91 Vasilissis Sophias Boulevard

Phones: 712951, 718401

**Hong Kong**

Hong Kong, 26 Garden Road

Phone: 239011

**Hungary**

Budapest, V. Szabadsag Ter 12

Phone: 329-375

**Iceland**

Reykjavik, Laufasvegur 21

Phone: 29100

**India**

New Delhi, Shanti Path, Chanakyapuri 21

Phone: 690351

**Iran**

Tehran, Talegani Avenue, P.O. Box 50 or Box 2000

Phones: 820-091, 824-001, 829-051

**Ireland**

Dublin, 42 Elgin Road, Ballsbridge

Phone: 688777

## Israel

Jerusalem, 18 Agron Road, Phone: 226312
Nablus Road, Phones: 282231, 272681

Tel Aviv, 71 Hayarkon Street
Phone: 54338

## Italy

Rome, Via V. Veneto 119/A
Phone: (06) 4674

Milan, Piazza Della Republica 32
Phones: (02) 652-841 through 652-845

Naples, Piazza della Republica, P.O. Box 18
Phone: (081) 660966

Florence, Lungarmo Amerigo Vespucci 38
Phone: (055) 298-276

## Jamaica

Kingston, Jamaica Mutual Life Center
2 Oxford Road, 3rd floor
Phone: 929-4850

## Japan

Tokyo, 10-1 Akasaka 1-chome, Minato-ku (107)
Phone: 583-7141

## Jordan

Amman, Jebel Amman, P.O. Box 354
Phones: 38930, 38724

## Kenya

Nairobi, Cotts House, Wabera Street
P.O. Box 30137
Phone: 334141

## Korea

Seoul, Sejong-Ro
Phones: 72-2601 through 72-2619

## Mexico

Mexico, D.F., Paseo de la Reforma 305
Phone: 553-3333

**Morocco**
Rabat, 2 Avenue de Marrakech,
P.O. Box 99, Phones: 30361, 30362
Casablanca, 8 Boulevard Moulay Youssef
P.O. Box 80, Phone: 22-41-49

**Nepal**
Kathmandu, Pani Pokhari
Phones: 11199, 12718, 11603, 11604

**Netherlands**
The Hague, 102 Longe Voorhout
Phone: 62-49-11

**New Zealand**
Wellington, 29 Firzherbert Terrace, Thorndon
P.O. Box 1190, Phone: 722-068

**Norway**
Oslo, Drammensveien 18, Oslo 1
Phones: 56-68-80

**Panama**
Panama, Avenida Balboa Y Calle 38
Apartado 6959, R.P. 5, Phone: Panama 25-3600

**Peru**
Lima, Corner Avenidas Inca Garcilaso de la Vega
and Espana, P.O. Box 1995, Phone: 286000

**Philippines**
Manila, 1201 Roxas Boulevard,
Phone: 598-011

**Poland**
Warsaw, Aleje Ujazdowskie 29/31
Phones: 283041 through 283049

**Portugal**
Lisbon, Avenida Duque de Louie No. 39
Phone: 570102

**Saudi Arabia**
Jidda, Palestine Road, Ruwais
Phones: 53410, 54110, 52188, 52396, 52589

## South Africa

Pretoria, Thibault House, 225 Pretorius Street
Phone: 48-4266

Capetown, Broadway Industries Center
Heerengracht, Foreshore, Phone: 021-471280

## Spain

Madrid, Serrano 75
Phones: 276-3400, 276-3600

## Sweden

Stockholm, Strandvagen 101
Phone: (08) 63-05-20

## Switzerland

Bern, Jubilaeumstrasse 93, 3005 Bern
Phone: (031) 430011

Zurich, Zollikerstrasse 141
Phone: 55-25-66

Geneva, 80 Rue du Lausanne
Phone: 32-70-20

## Turkey

Ankara, 110 Ataturk Boulevard
Phone: 26-54-70

Istanbul, 104-108 Mesrutiyet Caddesi, Tepebasi
Phones: 43-62-00, 43-62-09

## Union of Soviet Socialist Republics

Moskow, Ulitsa Chaykovskogo 19/21/23
Phones: 252-00-11 through 252-00-19

Leningrad, Petra Lavrova Street 15
P.O. Box L, Phone: 274-8235

## United Kingdom

London, England, 24/31 Grosvenor Square, W1A 1AE
Phone: (01) 499-9000

Belfast, Northern Ireland, Queen's House
14 Queen Street, BT1 6EQ
Phone: Belfast (0232) 28239

Edinburgh, Scotland, 3 Regent Terrace, EH7 5BW
Phone: 031-556-8315

## Venezuela

Caracas, Avenida Francisco de Miranda and
Avenida Principal de la Floresta
Phone: 284-7111

## Yugoslavia

Belgrade, Kneza Milosa 50
Phone: 645655

## Zaire

Kinshasa, 310 Avenue des Aviateurs
Phones: 25881 through 25886

---

# METRIC CONVERSION TABLES

### DISTANCES

| Kms | Miles |
|-----|-------|
| 1 | 5/8 |
| 2 | 1¼ |
| 3 | 2½ |
| 4 | 2⅞ |
| 5 | 3⅛ |
| 10 | 6¼ |
| 30 | 18⅝ |
| 50 | 31 |
| 100 | 62⅛ |
| 500 | 310¼ |

### MOTOR FUEL

| Liters | U.S. Gallons |
|--------|--------------|
| 1 | 0.26 |
| 5 | 1.32 |
| 10 | 2.64 |
| 20 | 5.28 |
| 100 | 26.42 |

### LIQUID

| Metric | U.S. Measures |
|--------|---------------|
| 1 liter | 1.06 quarts |
| .95 liters | 1 quart |
| 3.785 liters | 1 gallon |

### LENGTH

| Metric | U.S. Measures |
|--------|---------------|
| 2.54cm | 1 inch |
| .30m | 1 foot |
| .91m | 1 yard |
| 1.61 km | 1 mile |
| 1 meter | 1.093 yards |
| 1 meter | 3.281 feet |

### WEIGHT

| Metric | U.S. Measures |
|--------|---------------|
| 1 gram | .04 ounce |
| 1 kilogram | 2.2 pounds |
| 28.35 grams | 1 ounce |
| .45 kilograms | 1 pound |
| .91 metric tons | 1 ton |

# ACCESS INFORMATION IN OTHER COUNTRIES

## AUSTRALIA

HOBART

**HOBART FOR THE HANDICAPPED**, Tasmania Association of Disabled Persons, 20 Creek Road, Lenah Valley, Tasmania, Australia.

MELBOURNE

**MELBOURNE FOR THE HANDICAPPED**, by Ability Press and available from Victoria Association of Occupational Therapists, 24 Gold Road, South Oakleigh, Victoria 3167, Australia.
**MELBOURNE FOR THE HANDICAPPED**, Australian College of Occupational Therapists, 295 Queen Street, Melbourne, Victoria 3000, Australia.

PERTH

**GUIDE TO PERTH'S PICNIC SITES, PARKS AND OCEAN BEACHES FOR THOSE WITH RESTRICTED MOBILITY**, Community Recreation Council of Western Australia, Box 66, Wembly, Western Australia 6014, Australia.

SYDNEY *Australian Capitol Territory*

**SYDNEY FOR THE HANDICAPPED**, Australian Council for Rehabilitation for the Disabled, Action House, Edinburgh Avenue, Canberra City, A.C.T. 2601, Australia.

SYDNEY

**SYDNEY FOR THE HANDICAPPED**, Australian Council for Rehabilitation for the Disabled, Cleveland House, Bedford and Buckingham Street, Surrey Hills, Sydney N.S.W. Australia 2010, Australia.

TASMANIA

**HOLIDAY TOURS FOR THE HANDICAPPED:** *A Guide to Day Tours for the Handicapped in Southern Tasmania*, University of Tasmania, Faculty of Education, Special Education Department, G.P.O. Box 252c, Tasmania 7001, Australia.

NORTHEAST VICTORIA AND ALBURY FOR THE
HANDICAPPED, by the Border Morning Mail and available
from Occupational Therapy Department, Ovens and Murray
Hospital for the Aged, Beechworth, Victoria 3747, Australia.
VICTORIAN DISABLED MOTORISTS ASSOCIATION
ACCOMMODATIONS GUIDE, Victorian Disabled Motorists
Association, 3 Glencairn Avenue, Coburg, Victoria 3058,
Australia.

## BELGIUM

BATIMENTS ACCESSIBLES AUX HANDICAPES EN CHAISE
ROULANTE: BELGIQUE (Buildings Accessible to the
Handicapped in Wheelchairs: Belgium), Departement des
Aides Techniques, Croix Rouge de Belgique, 98 Chaussee de
Vleurgat, 1050 Bruxelles, Belgium. In French and English.
HOTELS 1979: BELGIQUE, BELGIE, BELGIEN, BELGIUM
(access indicated), Commissariat General du Tourisme, Rue
Marche aux Herbes 61, 1000 Bruxelles, Belgium; also from the
Belgian National Tourist Office, 745 Fifth Avenue, New York,
New York 10022. In French, English, Flemish, German, Italian
and Spanish.

## BERMUDA

HANDICAPPED VISITORS: FACILITIES IN BERMUDA,
Bermuda Department of Tourism, 630 Fifth Avenue, New
York, New York 10020; also from Richard Kitson, Society for
the Advancement of Travel for the Handicapped, P.O. Box 449,
Hamilton, Bermuda.

## CANADA

GUIDE FOR TRAVELING HEMOPHILIACS: DIRECTORY OF
NATIONAL TREATMENT CENTERS, by Abbott Laboratories
and available from World Federation of Hemophilia, 1170 Peel
Street, Room 1126, Montreal, Quebec H3B 2T4, Canada.
TRANSPORTATION IN CANADA: A GUIDE FOR THE
DISADVANTAGED, Transport Canada, Research and
Development Center, ATTN: Mrs. L. Suen, 100 Sherbrooke

Street West, Box 549, Place de L'Aviation, Montreal, Quebec H3A 2RS, Canada.

ALBERTA: EDMONTON

BUSINESS ACCESSIBILITY GUIDE FOR THE DISABLED IN EDMONTON, by Edmonton Social Services for the Disabled and available from Canadian Paraplegic Association, 302 Kingsway Garden Mall, 109th Street and Princess Elizabeth Avenue, Edmonton, Alberta T5G 3A6, Canada.

BRITISH COLUMBIA

BRITISH COLUMBIA TOURIST ACCOMMODATION DIRECTORY (access indicated), Ministry of Tourism and Small Business Development, 1117 Wharf Street, Victoria, British Columbia V8W 2Z2, Canada.

BROCKVILLE

REPORT FOR THE PHYSICALLY HANDICAPPED IN THE BROCKVILLE DOWNTOWN COMMERCIAL REGION, by Civil Engineering Technology students at St. Lawrence College and available from Ontario March of Dimes, 90 Thorncliffe Park Drive, Toronto, Ontario M4H 1M5, Canada.

BURLINGTON

AN ACCESSIBILITY GUIDEBOOK OF BURLINGTON, Burlington Social Planning Council, 386 Brant Street, Burlington, Ontario L7R 2E8, Canada.

CALGARY

GUIDE TO CALGARY FOR THE HANDICAPPED, Voluntary Bureau, 120-13 Avenue S.E., Calgary 21, Canada.

CAMBRIDGE

FREEWHEELING THROUGH CAMBRIDGE, by the Cambridge Committee for the Physically Disabled and available from Mrs. Jeanne Joslin, 61 Wentworth Avenue, Galt, Ontario N1S 1G8, Canada.

DRYDEN

A GUIDE FOR THE PHYSICALLY DISABLED AND THE ELDERLY IN THE DRYDEN AREA, by the Dryden Accessibility Survey Workers and available from Len Lotecki, Handicapped Action Group, c/o 18A Queen Street, Dryden, Ontario P8N 1A2, Canada.

**GUELPH**

AN ACCESSIBILITY GUIDEBOOK OF GUELPH, by the Architectural Barriers Committee and available from Ms. Mary DuQuensnay, St. Joseph's Hospital, Guelph, Ontario, Canada.

**HALIFAX-DARTMOUTH**

GUIDE FOR THE HANDICAPPED, The Canadian Paraplegic Association, 5599 Fenwick Street, Halifax, Nova Scotia B3H 1R2, Canada.

**KINGSTON**

A GUIDE TO KINGSTON FOR THE HANDICAPPED, Zonta Club of Kingston, 8 Birch Avenue, Kingston, Ontario, Canada.

**KITCHENER/WATERLOO**

AN ACCESSIBILITY GUIDE OF KITCHENER/WATERLOO, by Project Mobility and available from Mc Dean Mellway, Ontario March of Dimes, 877 Wilson Avenue, Kitchener, Ontario N2C 1J1, Canada.

**MONTREAL**

GUIDE FOR THE HANDICAPPED, Canadian Paraplegic Association, 153 Lyndhurst Avenue, Toronto 4, Canada.

**NEW BRUNSWICK**

MONCTON, FREDERICTON AND ST. JOHN, NEW BRUNSWICK, Multiple Sclerosis Society, Commerce House, 236 St. George Street, Room 204, Moncton, New Brunswick, Canada.

**NEWFOUNDLAND: ST. JOHN'S**

ACCESS: CITY OF ST. JOHN'S, Canadian Paraplegic Association, 21 Factory Lane, St. John's, Newfoundland A1C 6C4, Canada; also from The Hub, Box 4397, St. John's, Newfoundland A1C 6C4, Canada.

**NIAGARA FALLS**

NIAGARA FALLS: AN ACCESSIBILITY GUIDE FOR THE PHYSICALLY HANDICAPPED, Social Planning Council, 5017 Victoria Avenue, Niagara Falls, Ontario L2E 4C9, Canada.

NIAGARA FALLS: AN ACCESSIBILITY GUIDE FOR THE PHYSICALLY HANDICAPPED—RENTAL ACCOMMODATIONS, Social Planning Council, 5017 Victoria Avenue, Niagara Falls, Ontario L2E 4C9, Canada.

NIAGARA FALLS: AN ACCESSIBILITY GUIDE FOR THE PHYSICALLY HANDICAPPED—TOURIST FACILITIES, Social Planning Council, 5017 Victoria Avenue, Niagara Falls, Ontario L2E 4C9, Canada.

OAKVILLE

OAKVILLE WITH EASE, by the Rotary Club of Oakville and the Canadian General Electric Company and available from Rotary Club of Oakville, c/o T.H. Marshall, 56 Second Street, Oakville, Ontario L6J 3T2, Canada.

OTTAWA

OTTAWA: AN ACCESSIBILITY GUIDE, Rehabilitation Institute of Ottawa, 885 Meadowlands Drive, Room 403, Ottawa, Ontario K2C 3N2 Canada.

ACCESSIBILITY GUIDE: NATIONAL CAPITAL REGION, National Capital Commission, 48 Rideau Street, Ottawa, Ontario K1N 8K4, Canada.

PEEL

ACCESS TO PEEL REGION 1978, Peel Association for Handicapped Adults, Tonken Senior Public School, 3200 Tonken Road, Mississauga, Ontario L4Y 2Y6, Canada.

PETERBOROUGH

PETERBOROUGH GUIDE FOR THE PHYSICALLY HANDICAPPED, by the Rainbow Club of Peterborough and available from Disability Resource Center, St. Joseph's General Hospital, Peterborough, Ontario K9H 7B6, Canada.

QUEBEC

ACCÈS AUX LIEUX PUBLICS ("ACCESS TO PUBLIC PLACES"), Federation des Loires et Sports pour Handicapes du Quebec, Bureau R-12, 1415 E. Rue Jarry, Montreal, Quebec H2E 2Z7, Canada. In French.

QUEBEC IN A WHEELCHAIR, Henriette Germain, 1725 Rue Dunant, Sherbrooke, Quebec J1H 4A3, Canada. In English and French.

SASKATCHEWAN: SASKATOON

GUIDE TO SASKATOON FOR THE HANDICAPPED VISITOR, Canadian Paraplegic Association, 325 Fifth Avenue North, Saskatoon, Saskatchewan S7K 2P7, Canada.

A GUIDE FOR THE DISABLED: ST. CATHARINES, by St. Catharine's Standard and available from Niagara Peninsula Rehabilitation Centre, P.O. Box 924, St. Catharines, Ontario L2R 6Z4, Canada.

SAULT STE. MARIE
ACCESSIBILITY SAULT STE. MARIE, by Canada Works Program and available from Ontario March of Dimes, 180 Gore Street, Sault Ste. Marie, Ontario P6A 1M2, Canada.

SHERBROOKE
ACCESSIBILITY GUIDE FOR SHERBROOKE AND VICINITY, Guide de Quebec, ATTN: H. Germain, 1725 Rue Dunant, Sherbrooke, Quebec J1H 4A3, Canada. In English and French.

THUNDER BAY
ACCESSIBILITY GUIDE TO SPORTS AND RECREATIONAL FACILITIES FOR THE DISABLED, by Leisure Counseling and Recreational Activities for the Disabled and Available from Ability Centre, ATTN: Dr. Koivisto, 237 Camelot Street, Thunder Bay, Ontario P7A 4B2, Canada.

MINI GUIDE FOR THE HANDICAPPED VISITOR IN THUNDER BAY, by the Canada Works Project and available from Ability Center, ATTN: Dr. Koivisto, 237 Camelot Street, Thunder Bay, Ontario P7A 4B2, Canada.

TORONTO
ACCESSIBLE PLACES, Canadian Paraplegic Association, 520 Sutherland Drive, Toronto, Ontario M4G 3V9, Canada.

GUIDE TO APARTMENT LIVING FOR THE DISABLED IN METROPOLITAN TORONTO, by Housing Action for the Physically Handicapped and available from Ontario March of Dimes, 90 Thorncliffe Park Drive, Toronto, Ontario M4H 1M5, Canada.

GUIDE TO THE PHYSICAL ACCESSIBILITY OF THE UNIVERSITY OF TORONTO, by Opportunities Youth Grant and available from Ontario March of Dimes, 90 Thorncliffe Park Drive, Toronto, Ontario M4H 1M5, Canada.

TORONTO WITH EASE, The Canadian Paraplegic Association, 153 Lyndhurst Avenue, Toronto 4, Canada.

VANCOUVER

A GUIDE TO VANCOUVER FOR THE HANDICAPPED, Social Planning and Review Council of British Columbia, 1625 West 8th Avenue, Vancouver 9, BC Canada.

WATERLOO

ARRANGEMTNS FOR THE DISABLED AT THE UNIVERSITY OF WATERLOO, The University of Waterloo, Waterloo, Ontario, Canada.

WINDSOR/ESSEX COUNTY

AN ACCESSIBILITY GUIDE FOR THE PHYSICALLY HANDICAPPED: WINDSOR AND ESSEX COUNTY, by the Accessibility Committe and available from Ontario March of Dimes, Suite 410, Canada Trust Building, 176 University Avenue W., Windsor, Ontario N9A 5P1, Canada.

WINNIPEG

A GUIDE TO WINNIPEG FOR THE HANDICAPPED, The Canadian Paraplegic Association, Central Western Division, 825 Sherbrooke Street, Winnepeg 2, Manitoba, Canada.

YORK

SPOKES ACCESS GUIDE TO YORK REGION FOR THE DISABLED, Ontario March of Dimes, 90 Thorncliffe Park Drive, Toronto, Ontario M4H 1M5, Canada.

## DENMARK

HOTEL GUIDE FOR THE HANDICAPPED, Samfundet og Hjemmet for Vanfore, Borgervaenget 7, DK-2100, Copenhagen, Denmark. In Danish and English.

## ENGLAND

GARDENS TO VISIT (access indicated), Gardeners' Sunday White Witches, Claygate Road, Dorking, Surrey, England.

RADAR, Many access guides to cities in Great Britain are centrally available from the Royal Association for Disability and Rehabilitation (RADAR), 25 Mortimer Street, London W1N 8AB, England.

OUTINGS IN THE NORTHWEST FOR THE PHYSICALLY HANDICAPPED, Community Council of Lancashire, 15 Victoria Road, Fulwood, Preston PR2 4PS, England.

PROVIDING FOR DISABLED VISITORS, English Tourist Board, 4 Grosvenor Gardens, London SW1W ODU, England.

VISIT AN ENGLISH GARDEN, English Tourist Board, Marketing/Planning Research, 4 Grosvenor Gardens, London SW1W ODU, England.

WHERE TO STAY ... WHAT TO DO: A GUIDE TO SOUTHERN ENGLAND FOR THE DISABLED, Southern Tourist Board, Department TD, Old Town Hall, Leigh Road, Eastleigh, Hants SO5 4DE, England.

ACCESS TO PUBLIC CONVENIENCES (guide to toilets in England and Wales), available from RADAR.

BRITAIN FOR THE DISABLED, British Tourist Authority, 680 Fifth Avenue, New York, New York 10019.

BRITISH RAIL 1979: A GUIDE FOR DISABLED PEOPLE, available from RADAR.

DIRECTORY OF NATIONAL TREATMENT CENTRES (FOR TRAVELING HAEMOPHILIACS), the Haemophilia Society, P.O. Box 9, 16 Trinity Street, London SE1 1DE, England.

FERRY CONCESSIONS FOR THE DISABLED DRIVER, Disabled Drivers' Association, Ashwellthorpe Hall, Ashwellthorpe, Norwich, Norfolk NR15 1HP, England.

GOOD FOOD GUIDE 1979 (access indicated), Consumers' Association, Caxton Hill, Hertford SG13 7L2, England.

GUIDE TO FISHING FACILITIES FOR DISABLED ANGLERS, National Anglers' Council Officies, 5 Cowgate, Peterborough PE1 1LR, England.

HOLIDAYS: AN INFORMATION SHEET DESCRIBING THE DIFFERENT TYPES OF HOLIDAYS AVAILABLE FOR DISABLED PEOPLE, Greater London Association for the Disabled, 1 Thorpe Close, London W1O, England

LIST OF HOLIDAY FACILITIES IN THE UNITED KINGDOM, CHANNEL ISLANDS AND NORTHERN IRELAND, National Society for Mentally Handicapped Children, 117 Golden Lane, London EC1Y ORT, England.

MUSEUMS ASSOCIATION DATA SHEET: FACILITIES FOR

THE BLIND, Museums Association, 34 Bloomsbury Way, London W1A 2SF, England.

THEATRES AND CINEMAS, available from RADAR.

BAKEWELL

BAKEWELL, E.G. Hurfon, Hon. Secretary, Derbyshire Association for the Disabled, c/o Social Services Department, County Offices, Matlock, Derbyshire, England; also from A.W. Rose, Hon. Secretary, Derbyshire Association for the Disabled, Trentham House, Farley Hill, Matlock, Derbyshire, England.

BATH

BATH, by the Bath Association for the Disabled and available from Mrs. S. Dixon, Department of General Education, City of Bath Technical College, James Street West, Bath BA1 1UP, England.

BIRMINGHAM

BIRMINGHAM, by the Birmingham Voluntary Service Council, Birmingham, England, inconjunction with RADAR.

BRADFORD

BRADFORD, City of Bradford Welfare Department, 289 Rooley Lane, Bradford 5, Yorkshire, England.

BRIGHTON/HOVE

BRIGHTON AND HOVE: ACCESS GUIDE FOR THE DISABLED VISITOR, by Publications Ltd., and available from Brighton Voluntary Service Center, 17 Ditchling Rise, Brighton, East Sussex, England.

BURY ST. EDMONDS

BURY ST. EDMONDS, available from RADAR.

CAMBRIDGE

CAMBRIDGE, M.G. Martindale, Great Eastern House, Tenison Road, Cambridge, England; also from Mrs. J. Cobb, 86 DeFreville Avenue, Cambridge CB4 1HU, England.

CHESTNUT/WALTHAM CROSS

CHESTNUT/WALTHAM CROSS, available from RADAR.

CHICHESTER

CHICHESTER, by Outset and available from RADAR.

**COLCHESTER**

COLCHESTER, by the Totoract Club of Colchester, England.

**COVENTRY**

COVENTRY, available from RADAR.

**CROMER**

CROMER, available from RADAR.

**DONCASTER**

ACCESS TO DONCASTER, by the Doncaster Jubilee Social Club for the Disabled and the Community Resources Centre, Doncaster, England.

**DURHAM**

DURHAM, by the Durham Association for the Disabled, Durham, England, and available from RADAR.

**EXETER**

EXETER, Miss R.M. Habgood, Devonian Orthopaedic Association, 59 Wonford Road, Exeter, England.

**FYLDE COAST**

FYLDE COAST, by Fylde Coast Clubs of Lions International, Fylde Coast, England, and available from RADAR.

**GLOUCESTERSHIRE**

GLOUCESTERSHIRE, by the Gloucestershire Association for the Disabled, Gloucestershire, England.

**GREAT YARMOUTH**

GUIDE TO GREAT YARMOUTH, Great Yarmouth Association of Service Organizations, "Ferryside," High Road, Great Yarmouth, Norfolk, England.

**ISLE OF WIGHT**

HOLIDAYS WITH SAILING FACILITIES, Medina Valley Centre, Dodner Creek, Newport, Isle of Wight POL 5TE, England.

**KESWICK**

KESWICK, by the Allerdale Association for the Disabled, Keswick, England; and also Keswick-RADAR.

**KIDDERMINSTER**

KIDDERMINSTER, available from RADAR.

**LEEDS**

LEEDS FOR THE DISABLED, Access for the Disabled, 226

Stanningly Road, Leeds LS13 3BA, England; also from Mrs. Barbara Anderton, 31, The Grove, Alwoodley, Leeds LS17 7BN, England.

LONDON, Miss B.M. Stowe, Director, Disabled Living Foundation, Vincent House, Vincent Square, London SW1, England.

GUIDE TO LONDON'S UNDERGROUND STATIONS, available from RADAR.

LONDON FOR THE DISABLED, The British Travel Bookshop Ltd., 680 Fifth Avenue, New York, New York 10019.

WHO LOOKS AFTER YOU AT GATWICK AIRPORT? Airport Services, British airports Authority, 2 Buckingham Gate, London SW1E 6JL, England.

WHO LOOKS AFTER YOU AT HEATHROW AIRPORT? Airport Services, British Airports Authority, 2 Buckingham Gate, London SW1E 6JL, England.

WHO LOOKS AFTER YOU AT STANDSTED AIRPORT? Airport Services, British Airports Authority, 2 Buckingham Gate, London SW1E 6JL, England.

MANCHESTER, Manchester Youth and Community Service, Langton House, 82 Great Bridgewater Street, Manchester M1 5JY, England.

MANSFIELD, available from RADAR.

NEWCASTLE-UNDER-LYME, available from RADAR.

THE INS AND OUTS OF NEWCASTLE-UPON-TYNE, Newcastle-Upon-Tyne Council for the Disabled, M.E.A. House, Ellison Place, Newcastle-Upon-Tyne NE1 8XS, England.

NORTHAMPTON, the Council for Voluntary Service, Northampton, England.

**NORWICH**

NORWICH, City of Norwich Welfare Department, Regency House, Duke Street, Norwich, England.

**NOTTINGHAM**

NOTTINGHAM, the Nottingham Branch of the Chartered Society of Physiotherapy, Nottingham, England.

**OXFORD**

OXFORD, Miss A. Spokes, Organizing Secretary, Oxford Council of Social Services, City Chambers, Queen Street, Oxford OX1 1ES, England; also from RADAR.

**PAISLEY**

GUIDE TO PAISLEY, available from RADAR.

**PETERBOROUGH**

PETERBOROUGH, by the Peterborough Council for the Disabled, Peterborough, England, and available from RADAR.

**PLYMOUTH**

PLYMOUTH, by the Plymouth and District Disabled Fellowship, Plymouth, England.

**PORTSMOUTH**

PORTSMOUTH, by the Portsmouth Council of Community Service, Portsmouth, England.

**READING**

READING, by the pupils and ex-pupils of the Hephaistos School, Reading, England, and available from RADAR.

**SEVENOAKS**

SEVENOAKS, available from RADAR.

**SHEFFIELD**

SHEFFIELD by the Sheffield Coordinating Committee of the Disabled, Sheffield, England, and available from RADAR.

**SHREWSBURY**

SHREWSBURY, by the Shropshire Physically Handicapped Able-Bodied Organization and the West Midland Disabled Motorists Club, Shrewsbury, England.

**SOUTHWARK**

SOUTHWARK, by the Standing Committee for the Handicapped, Southwark, England.

ST. ALBANS

ST. ALBANS, by the St. Albans Guide for the Disabled Committee, St. Albans, England.

ST. HELENS

ST. HELENS, by the St. Helens Action Group for the Disabled, St. Helens, England.

STAFFORD

STAFFORD, available from RADAR.

STOKE-ON-TRENT

STOKE-ON-TRENT, available from RADAR.

TAUNTON

TAUNTON, by the Tauton and District Council of Social Services, Taunton, England.

TORBAY

TORBAY, by the Torbay Council of Social Services, Torbay, England, and available from RADAR

WIRRAL

WIRRAL, available from RADAR

WISBECH

WISBECH, by the Social Services Department, Wisbech, England.

WORCESTER

WORCESTER, available from RADAR.

AA GUIDE FOR THE DISABLED, Hotel and Information Services Department, Automobile Association, Account 7710/716, Fanum House, Basingstoke, Hants RG21 2EA, England.

ACCESS GUIDE TO THE NATURE RESERVES OF ENGLAND, SCOTLAND, AND WALES, available from RADAR.

### EUROPE in general

MOTEL GUIDE FOR THE DISABLED, European Highways, International Society for Rehabilitation of the Disabled, 219 East 44th Street, New York, New York 10017

### FRANCE

VACANCES POUR LES HANDICAPES (Vacations for the

Handicapped), Centre d'Information at de Documentation Jenunesse (C.I.D.J.), 101 Quai Branly, 75720 Paris, Cedex 15, France. In French.

ACCESS IN BRITTANY, Hephaistos School and St. Paul's School, England and available from *Rehabilitation/World*, Bookshelf Department, 20 West 40th Street, New York, New York 10018; also available from Gordon R. Couch, 68-B Castlebar Road, Ealing, London W5, England. In English.

ACCESS IN LOIRE, by the Hephaistos School and St. Paul's School, England and available from *Rehabilitation/World*, Bookshelf Department, 20 West 40th Street, New York, New York 10018; also available from Gordon R. Couch, 68-B Castlebar Road, Ealing, London W5, England. In English and French.

ACCESS IN PARIS, by the Hephaistos School and St. Paul's School, England and available from *Rehabilitation/World*, Bookshelf Department, 20 West 40th Street, New York, New York 10018; also available from Gordon R. Couch, 68-B Castlebar Road, Ealing, London W5, England. In English.

AEROPORT DE PARIS: GUIDE FOR DISABLED PERSONS, Paris Aeroport Authority, One World Trade Center, Suite 2551, New York, New York 10048 and also from: Aeroport de Paris, 291 Boulevard Respail, 75675 Paris, Cedex 14, France. In French and English.

## WEST GERMANY

AUTOBAHN SERVICE (access indicated), Gessellschaft fur Nebenbetriebe de Bundesautobahnan m.b.h., Poppelsdorfer Allee 24, 5300 Bonnl, Federal Republic of Germany. In German and English.

FERIENFUHRER ("Holiday Guide"), Bundesarbeitsgemeinschaft "Hilfe Fur Behinderte" e.V., Kirchfeldstrasse 149, 4 Dusseldorf, Federal Republic of Germany.

URLAUB, FERIEN, FREZEIT: KUREN UND ERHOLUNG FUR FAMLIIEN MIT BEHINDERTEN BZW. KRANKEN KINDERN UND JUGENDLICHEN ("Vacations, Holidays and Leisure: Cures and Relaxation for Families with Handicapped and Ill Children"), Bundesarbeitsgemeinschaft "Hilfe Fur Behinderte" e.V., Kirchfeldstrasse 149, 4 Dusseldorf, Federal Republic of Germany. In German.

DUSSELDORF

RAT + TAT + TIPS: WO FINDEN BEHINDERTE IN DUSSELDORF HILFE? ("Advice, Assistance and Tips: Where Can the Handicapped Find Help in Dusseldorf?"), Oberstadtdirektor der Landeshauptstadt Dusseldorf, Judgendamt Heinrich-Heine, Allee 53, 4 Dusseldorf, Federal Republic of Germany. In German.

FRANKFURT/MAIN

BEHINDERTEN-WEGWEISER: FRANKFURT/MAIN ("Guide for the Handicapped to Frankfurt/Main"), Kontaktstelle for Korperbehinderte and Langzeitkranke, Eschersheimer Landstrasse 567, 6000 Frankfurt Am Main 50, Federal Republic of Germany. In German.

HEIDELBERG

STADTFUHRER FUR BEHINDERTE HEIDELBERG ("Town Guide for the Handicapped to Heidelberg"), Gruppe '73: Initiative Korperbehinderte e.V., Postfach 102 448, D-6900 Heidelberg 1, Federal Republic of Germany. In German.

KOBLENZ

STADTFUHRER FUR BEHINDERTE DER STADT KOBLENZ ("Town Guide for the Handicapped to Koblenz"), "Der Kreis": Club Behinderter und ihrer Freunde e.V., Am Alten Hospital, 5400 Koblenz, Federal Republic of Germany. In German.

NECKARGEMUND

BEHINDERTENFUHRER NECKARGEMUND ("Access Guide to Neckargemund"), SPD-Ortsverein Neckargemund, Hollmuthstrasse 67, D-6903 Neckargemund, Federal Republic of Germany. In German.

BEHINDERTERFUHRER SCHLESWIG-HOLSTEIN ("Access Guide to Schleswig-Holstein"), Sozialministerium Schleswig-Holstein, Nrunswiker Strasse 16-22, 23 Kiel, Federal Republic of Germany. In German.

## IRELAND

DUBLIN

DUBLIN FOR THE DISABLED, Dr. Kevin P. O'Flanagan, Chairman, National Rehabilitation Board, 23 Upr. Fitzwilliam Street, Dublin, Ireland 61434

### IRELAND (NORTHERN)

HOLIDAY GUIDE FOR THE DISABLED: ACCESS GUIDE TO THIRTY-SIX PROVINCIAL TOWN AND BELFAST, Northern Ireland Committee for the Handicapped, Northern Ireland Council of Social Services, 2 Annadale Avenue, Belfast BT7 3JH, Northern Ireland, U.K.

COUNTY ANTRIM, available from RADAR.

COUNTY ARMAGH, available from RADAR.

COUNTY DOWN, available from RADAR.

COUNTY LONDONDERRY, available from RADAR.

COUNTY TYRONE & FERMANACH, available from RADAR.

BELFAST, available from RADAR.

## ITALY

ROME

ACCESS IN ROME, Open University Students' Association, Sherwood House, Sherwood Drive, Bletchley, Milton Keynes MK3 6HN, England.

HAVE WHEELS WILL TRAVEL: A STUDY TOUR OF ROME, Educational Explorers, 40 Silver Street, Reading RG1 2SU, England.

## ISRAEL

JERUSALEM

JERUSALEM: A GUIDE FOR THE HANDICAPPED, School of Occupational Therapy, Mount Scopus, Jerusalem, Israel. In Hebrew.

## JAPAN

ACCESSIBLE TOKYO, by the Tokyo Guidebook Committee and available from Mitsunobu Katsuya 3-12 Harue-cho, Edogawa-ku, Tokyo 132, Japan. In English.

## NETHERLANDS

HOLIDAY IN HOLLAND FOR THE HANDICAPPED, Netherlands National Tourist Office, Bezuidenhoutseweg 2, 2594 AV The Hague, Netherlands; also from Netherlands National Tourist Office, 576 Fifth Avenue, New York, New York 10036. In English.

MAP OF DAY RECREATION FACILITIES ACCESSIBLE FOR THE HANDICAPPED IN THE NETHERLANDS, Netherlands National Tourist Office, Bezuidenhoustseweg 2, 2594 AV The Hague, Netherlands. In Dutch.

AMSTERDAM

GUIDE FOR THE DISABLED TO AMSTERDAM, AVO Nederland, Centrale Administratie, P.O. Box 850, 3800 AW Amersfoort, The Netherlands. In Dutch.

## NEW ZEALAND

ACCESSIBLE ACCOMMODATIONS IN NEW ZEALAND, Public Relations Office, New Zealand Crippled Children Society, P.O. Box 6349, Te Aro, Wellington, New Zealand.

ACCESSIBLE PUBLIC TOILETS IN NEW ZEALAND, Public Relations Office, New Zealand Crippled Children Society, P.O. Box 6349, Te Aro, Wellington, New Zealand.

CHRISTCHURCH

A GUIDE TO CHRISTCHURCH FOR THE HANDICAPPED, Christchurch Coordinating Council for the Handicapped, Inc., P.O. Box 5234, Papanui, Christchurch, New Zealand; also available from Public Relations Office, P.O. Box 2600, Cnr. Oxford Terrace and Worcester Street, Christchurch, New Zealand.

NEW PLYMOUTH

ACCESS: A GUIDE FOR THE DISABLED, by the Jaycees, Pukekura Chapter and available from Public Relations Office, Liardet Street, New Plymouth, New Zealand.

## NORWAY

ACCESS IN NORWAY, by the Hephaistos School and St. Paul's School, England and available from *Rehabilitation/World*, Bookshelf Department, 20 West 40th Street, New York, New York 10018; also available from Gordon R. Couch, 68-B Castlebar Road, Ealing, London W5, England. In English.

HOTEL GUIDE FOR BEVEGELSESHEMMEDE, Norway Travel Association, H. Heyerdals gate 1, Oslo 1, Norway. In Norwegian.

## SCOTLAND

SCOTLAND FOR THE DISABLED: WHERE TO STAY, Edinburgh Committee for the Co-ordination of Service for the Disabled, Simon Square Centre, Howden Street, Edinburgh 8, Scotland.

ACCESSIBILITY IN THE CENTRAL REGION, Central Regional Council, Langgarth, Stirling FK8 2HA, Central Scotland, U.K.

ACCOMMODATIONS WITH FACILITIES FOR DISABLED VISITORS 1979, Scottish Tourist Board, 23 Ravelstone Terrace, Edinburgh EH4 3EU, Scotland, U.K.

GUIDE TO PUBLIC TOILETS IN SCOTLAND AND ACCESSIBLE TO PEOPLE IN WHEELCHAIRS, Scottish Council on Disability, 18/19 Claremont, Crescent, Edinburgh EH7 4QD, Scotland, U.K.

HOLIDAYS, Scottish Information Service for the Disabled, 18/19 Claremont, Crescent, Edinburgh EH7 4QD, Scotland, U.K.

HOLIDAYS FOR SPECIAL NEEDS 1979, Edinburgh Council of Social Service, Ainslie House, 11 Colme Street, Edinburgh EH3 6AG, Scotland, U.K.

HOLIDAYS WITH CARE IN SCOTLAND, Scottish Tourist Board, 23 Ravelstone Terrace, Edinburgh EH4 3EU, Scotland, U.K.

ABERDEEN

GUIDE TO ABERDEEN, Aberdeen Committee for the Welfare of the Disabled, 38 Castle Street, Aberdeen AB9 1AU, Scotland, U.K.

WHO LOOKS AFTER YOU AT ABERDEEN AIRPORT? Airport Services, British Airports Authority, 2 Buckingham Gate, London SW1E 6JL, England.

EDINBURGH/LOTHIAN

GUIDE TO EDINBURGH AND LOTHIAN FOR THE DISABLED, Edinburgh Committee for the Coordination of Services for the Disabled, Simon Square Center, Howden Street, Edinburgh EH8 9HW, Scotland, U.K.

WHO LOOKS AFTER YOU AT EDINBURGH AIRPORT? Airport Services, British Airports Authority, 2 Buckingham Gate, London SW1E 6JL, England.

GLASGOW

WHO LOOKS AFTER YOU AT GLASGOW AIRPORT? Airport Services, British Airports Authority, 2 Buckingham Gate, London SW1E 6JL, England.

PRESTWICK

WHO LOOKS AFTER YOU AT PRESTWICK AIRPORT? Airport Services, British Airports Authority, 2 Buckingham Gate, London·SW1E 6JL, England.

## SPAIN

BARCELONA

GUIA URBANA DE BARCELONA 1 - 1977, Federacion ECOM, Balmes 311, entl. 20, Barcelona 6, Spain. In Spanish.

## SWEDEN

HOMES OF RECREATION, The National Council for the Handicapped, Kungsgatan 48-I, S-11 35, Stockholm, Sweden. In English.

HOTELS, BOARDING HOUSES, ETC., AVAILABLE FOR PERSONS WHOSE ABILITY TO MOVE IS LIMITED, The National Council for the Handicapped, Kungsgatan 48-I, S-111 35, Stockholm, Sweden. In English.

HOTELS IN SWEDEN 1979 (access indicated), Swedish National Tourist Office, 75 Rockefeller Plaza, New York, New York 10019. In French, German and English.

INVESTIGATION AS REGARDS HOLIDAY VILLAGES, The National Council for the Handicapped, Kungsgatan 48-I, S-111 35, Stockholm, Sweden. In English.

HANDBOK FOR RORELSEHINDRADE: LINKOPING, by the Social Welfare Office and availble from Socialforvaltingen, Box 356, 581 03, Linkoping, Sweden. In Swedish.

MILJOGUIDE FOR OREBRO, Stadsarkitektkontoret, Orebro and is available from Plankontoret, Box 1425, 70114 Orebro, Sweden. In Swedish.

## SWITZERLAND

A GUIDE TO ACCESSIBLE MOTELS, CAMPSITES, YOUTH HOSTELS, RESTAURANTS AND TOILETS ALONG SWISS HIGHWAYS, Schweizerische Arbeitsgemeinschaft fur Korperbehinderte, Postfach 129, CH 8032, Zurich, Switzerland.

A HOLIDAY GUIDE FOR THE HANDICAPPED THROUGH SWITZERLAND (HOTELS, PENSIONS, APARTMENTS, ETC.), Schweizerische Arbeitsgemeinschaft fur Korperbehinderte, Postfach 129, CH 8032, Zurich, Switzerland.

SWISS HOTEL GUIDE FOR THE DISABLED, Swiss Invalid Association, Schweizerische Invaliden-Verband, Amthausquai 11, 4600 Olten 1, Switzerland. In English.

BASEL, Schweizerische Arbeitsgemeinschaft fur Korperbehinderte, Postfach 129, CH 8032, Zurich, Switzerland.

BERN, Schweizerische Arbeitsgemeinschaft fur Korperbehinderte, Postfach 129, CH 8032, Zurich, Switzerland. In German.

LAUSANNE Schweizerische Arbeitsgemeinschaft fur Korperbehinderte, Postfach 129, CH 8032, Zurich, Switzerland. In French.

LUCERNE, Schweizerische Arbeitsgemeinschaft fur Korperbehinderte, Postfach 129, CH 8032, Zurich, Switzerland. In German.

NEUCHATEL, Schweizerische Arbeitsgemeinschaft fur Korperbehinderte, Postfach 129, CH 8032, Zurich, Switzerland. In French.

ST. GALLEN, Schweizerische Arbeitsgemeinschaft fur Korperbehinderte, Postfach 129, CH 8032, Zurich, Switzerland.

ZURICH, Schweizerische Arbeitsgemeinschaft fur Korperbehinderte, Postfach 129, CH 8032, Zurich, Switzerland. In German.

SWITZERLAND—"SWISS HOTEL GUIDE FOR THE DISABLED," Swiss Invalid Association, Froburgstrasse 4, 4600 Olten, Switzerland.

## WALES

DISABLED VISITORS GUIDE TO WALES, Wales Council for the Disabled, Crescent Road, Caerphilly, Mid Glamorgan CF8 1XL, Wales, U.K.

LOCAL GUIDE TO WELSH TOWNS (Arfon District, Brecon, Cardiff, Colwyn, Llandudno, Neath, Prestatyn, Swansea), Wales Council for the Disabled, Crescent Road, Caerphilly, Mid Glamorgan CF8 1XL, Wales, U.K.

UNITED KINGDOM—ENGLAND—NORTHERN IRELAND—SCOTLAND—WALES: 1972 HOLIDAYS FOR THE PHYSICALLY HANDICAPPED, The Central Council for the Disabled, 34 Eccleston Square, London SW1V 1PE, England.

# FOREIGN EMBASSIES AND CONSULATES IN THE UNITED STATES

ARGENTINA
Office of the Embassy
1600 New Hampshire Avenue, N.W.
Washington, D.C. 20009
Phone: (202) 387-0705

AUSTRALIA
Office of the Embassy
1601 Massachusetts Avenue, N.W.
Washington, D.C. 20036
Phone: (202) 797-3000

AUSTRIA
Office of The Embassy
2343 Massachusetts Avenue, N.W.
Washington, D.C. 20008
Phone: (202) 483-4474

BAHAMAS (Commonwealth of the)
Office of the Embassy
Suite 865
600 New Hampshire Avenue, N.W.
Washington, D.C. 20037
Phone: (202) 338-3940

BARBADOS
Office of the Embassy
2144 Wyoming Avenue, N.W.
Washington, D.C. 20008
Phone (202) 387-7374

BELGIUM
Office of the Embassy
3330 Garfield Street
Washington, D.C. 20008
Phone: (202) 333-6900

BOLIVIA
Office of the Embassy
3014 Massachusetts Avenue, N.W.
Washington, D.C. 20036
Phone: (202) 483-4410

BRAZIL
Office of the Embassy
3006 Massachusetts Avenue, N.W.
Washington, D.C. 20008
Phone: (202) 797-0100

CANADA
Office of the Embassy
1746 Massachusetts Avenue, N.W.
Washington, D.C. 20036
Phone: (202) 785-1400

CHILE
Office of the Embassy
1732 Massachusetts Avenue, N.W.
Washington, D.C. 20036
Phone: (202) 785-1746

CHINA, People's Republic of
Office of the Embassy
2300 Connecticut Avenue, N.W.
Washington, D.C. 20008
Phone: (202) 797-9000

COLOMBIA
Office of the Embassy
2118 Leroy Place, N.W.
Washington, D.C. 20008
Phone: (202) 387-5828

CYPRUS
Office of the Embassy
2211 R Street, N.W.
Washington, D.C. 20008
Phone: (202) 462-5772

DENMARK
Office of the Embassy
3200 Whitehaven Street, N.W.
Washington, D.C. 20008
Phone: (202) 234-4300

ECUADOR
Office of the Embassy
2535 Fifteenth Street, N.W.
Washington, D.C. 20009
Phone: (202) 234-7200

EGYPT
Office of the Embassy
2310 Decatur Place, N.W.
Washington, D.C. 20008
Phone: (202) 232-5400

FINLAND
Office of the Embassy
1900 Twenty-Fourth Street, N.W.
Washington, D.C. 20008
Phone: (202) 462-0556

FRANCE
Office of the Embassy
2535 Belmont Road, N.W.
Washington, D.C. 20008
Phone: (202) 234-0990

GREECE
Office of the Embassy
2221 Massachusetts Avenue, N.W.
Washington, D.C. 20008
Phone: (202) 667-3168

GUATEMALA
Office of the Embassy
2220 R Street, N.W.
Washington, D.C. 20008
Phone: (202) 332-2865

HAITI
Office of the Embassy
4400 Seventeenth Street, N.W.
Washington, D.C. 20011
Phone: (202) 723-7000

ICELAND
Office of the Embassy
2022 Connecticut Avenue, N.W.
Washington, D.C. 20008
Phone: (202) 265-6653

IRELAND
Office of the Embassy
2234 Massachusetts Avenue, N.W.
Washington, D.C. 20008
Phone: (202) 483-7639

ISRAEL
Office of the Embassy
1621 Twenty-second Street, N.W.
Washington, D.C. 20008
Phone: (202) 483-4100

ITALY
Office of the Embassy
1601 Fuller Street, N.W.
Washington, D.C. 20009
Phone: (202) 234-1935

JAMAICA
Office of the Embassy
1666 Connecticut Avenue, N.W.
Washington, D.C. 20009
Phone: (202) 387-1010

JAPAN
Office of the Embassy
2520 Massachusetts Avenue, N.W.
Washington, D.C. 20008
Phone: (202) 234-2266

KENYA
Office of the Embassy
2249 R Street, N.W.
Washington, D.C. 20008
Phone: (202) 387-6101

LITHUANIA
Office of the Embassy
2622 Sixteenth Street, N.W.
Washington, D.C. 20009
Phone: (202) 234-5860

LUXEMBOURG
Office of the Embassy
2200 Massachusetts Avenue, N.W.
Washington, D.C. 20008
Phone: (202) 265-4171

MEXICO
Office of the Embassy
2829 Sixteenth Street, N.W.
Washington, D.C. 20009
Phone: (202) 234-6000

MOROCCO
Office of the Embassy
1601 Twenty-first Street, N.W.
Washington, D.C. 20009
Phone: (202) 462-7979

NETHERLANDS
Office of the Embassy
4200 Linnean Avenue, N.W.
Washington, D.C. 20008
Phone: (202) 244-5300

NEW ZEALAND
Office of the Embassy
19 Observatory Circle, N.W.
Washington, D.C. 20008
Phone: (202) 265-1721

NORWAY
Office of the Embassy
2720 Thirty-fourth Street, N.W.
Washington, D.C. 20008
Phone: (202) 333-6000

PANAMA
Office of the Embassy
2862 McGill Terrace, N.W.
Washington, D.C. 20008
Phone: (202) 483-1407

PERU
Office of the Embassy
1700 Massachusetts Avenue, N.W.
Washington, D.C. 20036
Phone: (202) 833-9860

PHILIPPINES
Office of the Embassy
1617 Massachusetts Avenue, N.W.
Washington, D.C. 20036
Phone: (202) 483-1414

POLAND
Office of the Embassy
2640 Sixteenth Street, N.W.
Washington, D.C. 20009
Phone: (202) 234-3800

PORTUGAL
Office of the Embassy
2125 Kalorama Road, N.W.
Washington, D.C. 20008
Phone: (202) 265-1643

SINGAPORE
Office of the Embassy
1824 R Street, N.W.
Washington, D.C. 20009
Phone: (202) 667-7555

SOUTH AFRICA
Office of the Embassy
3051 Massachusetts Avenue, N.W.
Washington, D.C. 20008
Phone: (202) 232-4400

SPAIN
Office of the Embassy
2700 Fifteenth Street, N.W.
Washington, D.C. 20009
Phone: (202) 265-0190

SWEDEN
Office of the Embassy
Suite 1200
600 New Hampshire Avenue, N.W.
Washington, D.C. 20037
Phone: (202) 965-4100

SWITZERLAND
Office of the Embassy
2900 Cathedral Avenue, N.W.
Washington, D.C. 20008
Phone: (202) 462-1811

SYRIA
Office of the Embassy
2215 Wyoming Avenue, N.W.
Washington, D.C. 20008
Phone: (202) 232-6313

TURKEY
Office of the Embassy
1606 Twenty-third Street, N.W.
Washington, D.C. 20008
Phone: (202) 667-6400

UNION OF SOVIET
SOCIALIST REPUBLICS
Office of the Embassy
1125 Sixteenth Street, N.W.
Washington, D.C. 20036
Phone: (202) 628-7551

UNITED KINGDOM
Office of the Embassy
3100 Massachussetts Avenue, N.W.
Washington, D.C. 20008
Phone: (202) 462-1340

VENEZUELA
Office of the Embassy
2445 Massachusetts Avenue, N.W.
Washington, D.C. 20008
Phone: (202) 265-9600

ZAIRE
Office of the Embassy
1800 New Hampshire Avenue, N.W.
Washington, D.C. 20009
Phone: (202) 234-7690

# HOTEL/MOTEL CHAINS WITH ACCESSIBLE UNITS IN THE UNITED STATES

DOWNTOWNER/ROWNTOWNER INNS
   for accessibility information call 1-800-238-6161
   The Directory of Inns is available from
   Hotel Systems of America, Inc.
   Box 171807
   Memphis, Tennessee 38117

HOLIDAY INN DIRECTORY—WORLDWIDE (access indicated)
   Holiday Inns, Inc., Public Relations Hotel Group
   3796 Lamar Avenue
   Memphis, Tennessee 38118

MARRIOTT HOTELS DIRECTORY (access indicated)
   Marriott Corporation, Marriott Drive
   Washington, D.C. 20058

RAMADA INNS DIRECTORY (access indicated)
   Ramada Inns, Inc., Box 590-JH
   Phoenix, Arizona 85001

RODEWAY INNS DIRECTORY (access indicated)
   Rodeway Inns of America
   2525 Stemmons Freeway, Suite 800
   Dallas, Texas 75207

TRAVELODGE DIRECTORY (access indicated)
   Travelodge Directory
   250 Travelodge Drive
   El Cajon, California 92090

WESTERN INTERNATIONAL HOTEL
 FACILITIES FOR THE HANDICAPPED
   Western International Hotels
   2000 Fifth Avenue
   Seattle, Washington 98121

# MEDICAL ASSISTANCE FOR TRAVELERS

INTERNATIONAL SOS ASSISTANCE, 2 Neshaminy Interplex
Trevose, PA 19047   *800* 523-8930

HEALTH CARE ABROAD, 1029 Investment Building
1511 K Street, N.W., Washington, D.C. 20005   *800* 336-3310

MEDIC ALERT, P.O. Box 1009
Turlock, CA 95381   *800* 344-3226

REHABILITATION INTERNATIONAL/USA, 20 West 40th Street
New York, NY 10018   *212* 869-9907

TRAVEL INFORMATION CENTER
MOSS REHABILITATION HOSPITAL
12 Street and Tabor Road
Philadelphia, PA 19131   *212* 329-5715

SATH—SOCIETY FOR THE ADVANCEMENT OF
TRAVEL FOR THE HANDICAPPED
26 Court Street, Brooklyn, NY 11242

INTERMEDIC, 777 Third Avenue
New York, NY 10017   *212* 486-8974

TRAVEL INFORMATION/REHABILITATION
RESEARCH AND TRAINING CENTER
George Washington University Medical Center
1828 L Street, N.W., Suite 704
Washington, D.C. 20036   *202* 676-4819

THE EASTER SEAL SOCIETY, 2 Park Avenue, Suite 1815
New York, NY 10016

EPILEPSY FOUNDATION OF AMERICA
1828 L Street, N.W., Washington, D.C. 20036

INTERNATIONAL ASSOCIATION OF MEDICAL ASSISTANCE
FOR TRAVELERS (IAMAT)
350 Fifth Avenue, New York, NY 10001

VACATIONING WITH DIABETES, Squibb Public Affairs
P.O. Box 4000, Princeton, NJ 08540

WHERE TURNING WHEELS STOP, Paralyzed Veterans
of America, 3636 16th Street, N.W., Washington, D.C. 20010

GUIDE FOR TRAVELING HEMOPHILIACS/DIRECTORY
OF NATIONAL TREATMENT CENTERS
World Federation of Hemophiliacs, 1170 Peel Street
Room 1126, Montreal, Quebec H3B 2T4, Canada

TRAVEL FOR THE PATIENT WITH CHRONIC
OBSTRUCTIVE PULMONARY DISEASE
Rehabilitation Research and Training Center
George Washington University Medical Center, Ross Hall
Room 714, 2300 I Street, N.W., Washington, D.C. 20037

DIALYSIS WORLDWIDE FOR THE TRAVELING PATIENT
(NAPHY), 505 Northern Boulevard, Great Neck, NY 11021

---

## PUBLICATIONS FROM FEDERAL SOURCES FOR HANDICAPPED TRAVELERS

ACCESS NATIONAL PARKS: A GUIDE FOR HANDICAPPED
VISITORS, prepared in 1978, 197 pages, and available for $3.50
from: Superintendent of Documents
U.S. Government Printing Office, Washington, D.C. 20402
GPO Stock Number 024-005-00691-5.

ACCESS TRAVEL: A GUIDE TO THE ACCESSIBILITY OF AIR-
PORT TERMINALS, a leaflet prepared in 1979 and available
free from: Consumer Information Center
Pueblo, Colorado 81009.

AIR TRANSPORTATION OF HANDICAPPED PERSONS, a cir-
cular prepared in 1977 and available free from:
Federal Aviation Administration, APA 400
800 Independence Avenue
S.W., Washington, D.C. 20591.

ASSISTING THE WHEELCHAIR TRAVELER, a pamphlet prepared in 1980 and available free from:
Office of Human Development Services—
Printing and Distribution, Room 318D, Humphrey Building
200 Independence Avenue, S.W.
Washington, D.C. 20201.

HANDICAPPED ACCESS AND HISTORIC PRESERVATION
prepared in 1978 and available free from:
HCRS Information Exchange, Division of P.A.R.T.S.
440 G Street, N.W.
Washington, D.C. 20243.

HIGHWAY REST AREAS FOR HANDICAPPED TRAVELERS
prepared in 1980 and available free from: President's
Committee on Employment of the Handicapped
111 20th Street, N.W.
Room 606, Washington, D.C. 20036.

SMITHSONIAN: A GUIDE FOR DISABLED PEOPLE, prepared
in 1980, 25 pages, and available free from: President's
Committee on Employment of the Handicapped, (see above).

THE YELLOW BOOK: HEALTH INFORMATION FOR INTERNATIONAL TRAVEL, available from: U.S. Department of
Health and Human Services, Center for Disease Control
Atlanta, Georgia 30333.

# TOUR OPERATORS WHO SPECIALIZE IN TOURS FOR THE DISABLED

ACCESSIBLE ADVENTURES, INC.
1050 Brownlee Road, P.O. Box 16137, Memphis, TN 38116

ALL STATE TOURS, 26 Court Street, Brooklyn, NY 11242

BOSWELL AND JOHNSON TRAVEL SERVICE (ENGLAND)
80 Grosvenor Street, London W1, England

CLARK TOURS—GUATEMALA FOR THE HANDICAPPED
331 Madison Avenue, Suite 1007, New York, NY 10017

DIALYSIS IN WONDERLAND
Division of Artificial Organs
Dumke Building, University of Utah—Salt Lake City, UT 841

EVERGREEN TRAVEL
R9505L 44th Avenue West, Lynwood, WA 98036

FLYING WHEELS TRAVEL
143 West Bridge, P.O. Box 382, Owatonna, MN 55060

THE HANDICAPPED, 26 Court Street, Brooklyn, NY 11242

HANDY-CAP HORIZONS
3250 East Loretta Drive, Indianapolis, IN 46227

HELPING HANDS TOURS
175 Fifth Avenue, New York, NY 10010

ISLAND HOLIDAYS
214 Grant Avenue, San Francisco, CA 94108

MONTE TOURS, 347 Fifth Avenue, New York, NY 10016

NEW FREEDOM ADVENTURES
2684 Nostrand Avenue, Brooklyn, NY 11210

NEW HORIZONS
Post Office Box 652, Belmont, MA 02178

RAMBLING TOURS, P.O. Box 1304, Hallandale, FL 33009

S.C.I.L.L.S. TOURS AND TRAVEL
(Specialized Challenges in Leisure Lifestyles)
2000 Barney Ave., Menlo Park, CA 94025

SATH—SOCIETY FOR THE ADVANCEMENT OF TRAVEL FOR
TOURIST PROMOTION (SCOTLAND)
36 Castle Street, Edinburgh EH2 3BN, Scotland

WHOLE PERSON TOURS
P.O. Box 1084, Bayonne, NJ 07002

WILDERNESS ENCOUNTERS, INC.
693 West Grand River, Okemos, MI 48864

WINGS ON WHEELS
19505 44th Street West, Lynwood, WA 98036

WORLDWAYS—HAWAIIAN HOLIDAYS
711 Third Avenue, New York, NY 10017

## CURRENCY

| | |
|---:|:---|
| ARGENTINA | 100 centavos = 1 peso |
| AUSTRIA | 100 groschen = 1 schilling |
| BELGIUM | 100 centimes = 1 franc |
| BRAZIL | 100 centavos = 1 cruzeiro |
| CHINA | 100 fen = 1 yuan |
| DENMARK | 100 ore = 1 krone |
| FINLAND | 100 penni = 1 markka |
| FRANCE | 100 centimes = 1 franc |
| WEST GERMANY | 100 pfennige = 1 deutsche mark |
| GREECE | 100 lepta = 1 drachma |
| ISRAEL | 100 agorot = 1 pound |
| ITALY | 100 centesimi = 1 lira |
| JAPAN | 100 sen = 1 yen |
| MEXICO | 100 centavos = 1 peso |
| PORTUGAL | 100 centavos = 1 escudo |
| SPAIN | 100 centimos = 1 peseta |
| SWEDEN | 100 ore = 1 krona |
| U.S.S.R. | 100 kopecks = 1 ruble |
| UNITED KINGDOM | 100 pence = 1 pound |
| UNITED STATES | 100 cents = 1 dollar |

# CLOTHING SIZES

| SHOES | | | WOMEN | | | MEN | | |
|---|---|---|---|---|---|---|---|---|
| American | | 4½ | 6½ | 8½ | 10½ | 8½ | 10½ | 12½ |
| British | | 3 | 5 | 7 | 9 | 7 | 9 | 11 |
| Continental/Metric | | 36 | 38 | 40 | 42 | 41 | 43 | 45 |

| MEN'S SHIRTS | | | | | | | | |
|---|---|---|---|---|---|---|---|---|
| British/American | 13½ | 14 | 14½ | 15 | 15½ | 16 | 16½ | 17 |
| Continental/Metric | 34 | 36 | 37 | 38 | 39 | 41 | 42 | 43 |

| MEN'S SUITS | | | | | | | |
|---|---|---|---|---|---|---|---|
| American | 34 | 36 | 38 | 40 | 42 | 44 | 46 |
| Metric | 44 | 46 | 48 | 50 | 52 | 54 | 56 |

| WOMEN'S COATS/DRESSES | | | | | | | |
|---|---|---|---|---|---|---|---|
| American | 8 | 10 | 12 | 14 | 16 | 18 | 20 |
| Metric | 36 | 38 | 40 | 42 | 44 | 46 | 48 |

| WOMEN'S SWEATERS | | | | | | | |
|---|---|---|---|---|---|---|---|
| American | 32 | 34 | 36 | 38 | 40 | 42 | 44 |
| Metric | 40 | 42 | 44 | 46 | 48 | 50 | 52 |

| STOCKINGS | | | | | | | |
|---|---|---|---|---|---|---|---|
| American | 8 | 8½ | 9 | 9½ | 10 | 10½ | 11 |
| Metric | 0 | 1 | 2 | 3 | 4 | 5 | 6 |

| HATS | | | | | |
|---|---|---|---|---|---|
| American | 6¼ | 6⅜ | 6½ | 6¾ | 7 |
| Measuring around the crown of the head | 20¼ | 20½ | 20⅞ | 21⅝ | 22 |

| CHILDREN'S DRESSES/COATS | | | | | |
|---|---|---|---|---|---|
| American | 2 | 4 | 6 | 8 | 10 |
| Continental/Metric | 2 | 3 | 5 | 7 | 9 |

| JUNIOR MISSES DRESSES/COATS | | | | |
|---|---|---|---|---|
| American | 8 | 10 | 13 | 15 |
| Continental/Metric | 7 | 9 | 10 | 12 |

# VISAS AND PASSPORTS

Information on visa requirements change frequently. Check, before travelling, with the Consular officials of the countries you plan to visit.

| COUNTRY | CURRENT STATUS |
|---|---|
| ARGENTINA | Passport required. Tourist visa not required up to three months. |
| AUSTRALIA | Passport required. Transit visa not required up to 72 hours. |
| AUSTRIA | Passport required. Visa not required up to three months. |
| BAHAMAS | No passport required. No visa required. |
| BELGIUM | Passport required. No visa required for 90 days. |
| BERMUDA | No passport required. No visa required. |
| BRAZIL | Passport required. No visa required for 90 days. |
| CANADA | No passport required. No visa required. |
| CHINA, PEOPLE'S REPUBLIC OF | Passport required. Visa required in advance. |
| DENMARK | Passport required. Visa not required for three months. |
| EGYPT | Passport required. Visa required. |
| FINLAND | Passport required. Visa not required for three months. |
| FRANCE | Passport required. Visa not required for three months |

| | |
|---|---|
| GERMANY, WEST | Passport required. Visa not required for three months. |
| GREECE | Passport required. Visa not required for two months. |
| HONG KONG | Passport required. Visa not required for one month. |
| INDIA | Passport required. Transit visa required. |
| IRELAND | Passport required. No visa required. |
| ISRAEL | Passport required. No visa required for three months. |
| ITALY | Passport required. Visa not required up to three months. |
| JAPAN | Passport required. Visa required. |
| MEXICO | Passport not required. Visa not required. |
| NORWAY | Passport required. Visa not required for three months. |
| PORTUGAL | Passport required. Visa not required for up to 60 days. |
| SINGAPORE | Passport required. Visa required. |
| SPAIN | Passport required. Visa not required for six months. |
| SWEDEN | Passport required. Visa not required up to three months. |
| SWITZERLAND | Passport required. Visa not required up to three months. |
| TURKEY | Passport required. Visa not required up to three months. |
| UNION OF SOVIET SOCIALIST REPUBLICS | Passport required. Visa required. |
| UNITED KINGDOM | Passport required. Visa not required. |
| VENEZUELA | Passport required. Visa required. |
| YUGOSLAVIA | Passport required. Visa required. |
| ZAMBIA | Passport required. Transit visa required. |

| WEATHER CONDITIONS AROUND THE WORLD | | | | | Temperature Extremes | | Annual Rainfall |
|---|---|---|---|---|---|---|---|
| COUNTRY | JAN. | APR. | JULY | OCT. | HIGH | LOW | in inches |
| Australia | 55–82 | 44–67 | 33–52 | 43–68 | 109 | 14 | 23.0 |
| Austria | 26–34 | 41–57 | 59–75 | 44–55 | 98 | −14 | 25.6 |
| Bulgaria | 22–34 | 41–62 | 57–82 | 42–63 | 99 | −17 | 25.0 |
| China (Peking) | 49–65 | 65–77 | 77–91 | 67–85 | 101 | 31 | 63.6 |
| Cyprus | 42–58 | 50–74 | 69–97 | 58–81 | 116 | 23 | 14.6 |
| Czechoslovakia | 25–34 | 40–55 | 58–74 | 44–54 | 98 | −16 | 19.3 |
| Denmark | 29–36 | 37–50 | 55–72 | 42–53 | 91 | −3 | 23.3 |
| England | 35–44 | 40–56 | 55–73 | 44–58 | 99 | 9 | 22.9 |
| Finland | 17–27 | 31–43 | 57–71 | 37–45 | 89 | −23 | 27.6 |
| France | 32–42 | 41–60 | 55–76 | 44–59 | 105 | 1 | 22.3 |
| Germany (West) | 28–35 | 39–51 | 59–69 | 44–53 | 92 | −4 | 28.9 |
| Greece | 42–54 | 52–67 | 72–90 | 60–74 | 109 | 20 | 15.8 |
| Hungary | 26–35 | 44–62 | 61–82 | 45–61 | 103 | −10 | 24.2 |
| Iceland | 28–36 | 33–43 | 48–58 | 36–44 | 74 | 4 | 33.9 |
| Iraq | 39–60 | 57–85 | 76–110 | 61–92 | 121 | 18 | 5.5 |
| Ireland | 35–47 | 38–54 | 51–67 | 43–57 | 86 | 8 | 29.7 |
| Israel | 41–55 | 50–73 | 63–87 | 59–81 | 107 | 26 | 19.7 |
| Italy | 39–54 | 46–68 | 53–73 | 53–73 | 104 | 20 | 29.5 |

| COUNTRY | JAN. | APR. | JULY | OCT. | Temperature Extremes HIGH | LOW | Annual Rainfall in inches |
|---|---|---|---|---|---|---|---|
| Japan | 29–47 | 46–63 | 70–83 | 55–69 | 101 | 17 | 61.6 |
| Malta | 51–59 | 56–66 | 72–84 | 66–76 | 105 | 34 | 20.3 |
| Morocco | 46–63 | 52–71 | 63–82 | 58–77 | 118 | 32 | 19.8 |
| Netherlands | 34–40 | 43–52 | 59–69 | 48–56 | 95 | 3 | 25.6 |
| Norway | 20–30 | 34 50 | 56–73 | 37–49 | 93 | −21 | 26.9 |
| Peru | 66 82 | 63–80 | 57–67 | 58–71 | 98 | 49 | 1.6 |
| Poland | 21–30 | 38–54 | 56–75 | 41 51 | 90 | −22 | 22.0 |
| Portugal | 46–56 | 52–64 | 63–79 | 57–69 | 103 | 29 | 27.0 |
| Romania | 20–33 | 41–63 | 61–86 | 44–65 | 105 | −18 | 22.8 |
| Spain | 33–47 | 44–64 | 62–87 | 48–66 | 102 | 14 | 16.5 |
| Sweden | 23–31 | 32–45 | 55–70 | 39–48 | 97 | −26 | 22.4 |
| Switzerland | 26–35 | 39–56 | 56–74 | 42–55 | 96 | −9 | 38.5 |
| Thailand | 67–89 | 78–95 | 76–90 | 76–88 | 104 | 50 | 57.8 |
| Turkey | 36–45 | 45–61 | 65–81 | 54–67 | 100 | 17 | 31.5 |
| U.S.S.R. | 9–21 | 31–47 | 55–78 | 34–46 | 96 | −27 | 24.8 |
| Venezuela | 56–75 | 60–81 | 61–78 | 61–79 | 91 | 45 | 32.9 |
| Yugoslavia | 27–37 | 45–64 | 61–84 | 47–65 | 107 | −14 | 24.6 |

Source: Reader's Digest 1980 Almanac and Yearbook     Reader's Digest Association, Pleasantville, New York 10570

# TOURIST VOCABULARY TIPS

If you find you have difficulty with foreign languages, write each of the necessary vocabulary words on 3 x 5 index cards. Instead of struggling with a strange language or pronunciation in a time of stress, just take out the appropriate card and show it to someone who can help. Write both the foreign language and the English translation on the same side of the card. Take some blank cards with you so that someone can write phrases or directions for you.

## TOURIST VOCABULARY

| ENGLISH | DANISH | GREEK |
|---|---|---|
| 1. Good Morning | 1. God Morgen | 1. Kalimera |
| 2. Good Evening | 2. God Aften | 2. Kalispera |
| 3. Goodbye | 3. Farvel | 3. Kalf andamosi |
| 4. How much does this cost? | 4. Hvor meget kosterden? | 4. Posso kani? |
| 5. Many thanks | 5. Tak | 5. Efchoristo |
| 6. I am ill | 6. Jeg er syd | 6. Eme arostos |
| 7. I want a doctor | 7. Kunt U mij dichtst bijzijnde wijzen de dokter | 7. Kahlehsteh ehnah yeeahtro greegorah |
| 8. Where is the bathroom? | 8. badevoerelse | 8. banio |
| 9. Please | 9. voer sa venlig | 9. Parakalo |
| 10. Ambulance | 10. ambulance | 10. Nosokomiako |
| 11. Yes | 11. Ja | 11. neh |
| 12. No | 12. Nej | 12. okhee |
| 13. I am disabled | 13. Ek hebeen gehandicapte | 13. Eme anapiros |
| 14. I would like to buy | 14. Var kanjag kopa | 14. Tha fthela no agorasso |
| 15. The menu, please. | 15. me jeg se spise-kortet? | 15. dos mou ton katalogo? |
| 16. The bill, please | 16. Jeg vil gerne betale | 16. To logariasmo |
| 17. Police station | 17. Politiet | 17. Asstinomiko tmima |
| 18. What time is it? | 18. Hvad er klokken? | 18. Ti'ora ine? |
| 19. Ladies | 19. Damer | 19. Kirfa |
| 20. Gentlemen | 20. Herrer | 20. Kfrie |

| ENGLISH | GERMAN | FRENCH |
|---|---|---|
| 1. Good Morning | 1. Guten morgen | 1. Bonjour |
| 2. Good Evening | 2. Guten abend | 2. Bon soir |
| 3. Goodbye | 3. Guten tag | 3. Au revoir |
| 4. How much does this cost? | 4. Was kostet das? | 4. Combien? |
| 5. Many thanks | 5. Vielen Dank | 5. Merci beaucoup |
| 6. I am ill | 6. Ich bin krank | 6. Je suis malade |
| 7. I want a doctor | 7. Ich brauche einen doktor | 7. Je desire consulter un medecin |
| 0. Where is the bathroom? | 8. Wo ist das badezimmer? | 8. Où est la salle de bain? |
| 9. Please | 9. Bitte | 9. S'il vous plaît |
| 10. Ambulance | 10. Krankenwagen | 10. Appelez un ambulance |
| 11. Yes | 11. Ja | 11. Oui |
| 12. No | 12. Nein | 12. Non |
| 13. I am disabled | 13. Ich bin körperbehinderte | 13. Je suis infirme |
| 14. I would like to buy | 14. Ich möchte kaufen | 14. Je desire acheter |
| 15. The menu, please | 15. Die speiskarte, bitte? | 15. Donnez-nous la carte, s'il vous plaît |
| 16. The bill, please | 16. Jeg vil gerne betale | 16. L'addition, sil vous plait |
| 17. Police station | 17. die Polizei | 17. Ou est la gendarmerie (la police) |
| 18. What time is it? | 18. Wieviel uhr ist es? | 18. Quel heure est-il? |
| 19. Ladies | 19. Damen | 19. Dames |
| 20. Gentlemen | 20. Herren | 20. Messieurs |

| ENGLISH | POLISH | ITALIAN |
|---|---|---|
| 1. Good Morning | 1. Dzien dobry | 1. Buongiorno |
| 2. Good Evening | 2. Dobry wieczor | 2. Buona sera |
| 3. Goodbye | 3. Do widzenia | 3. Ciao, arrivederci |
| 4. How much does this cost? | 4. Ile? | 4. Quanto costa? |
| 5. Many thanks | 5. Dziekuje | 5. Grazie |
| 6. I am ill | 6. Ja jestem chori | 6. Mi sento male; Non mi sento bene |
| 7. I want a doctor | 7. Prosze wezwac le karza | 7. Dove si trova il medico |
| 8. Where is the bathroom? | 8. Gdzie jest toaleta? | 8. Dove si trova il gabinetto? |
| 9. Please | 9. Prosze | 9. Per favore |
| 10. Ambulance | 10. Prosze wezwac pogotowie | 10. L'ambulanza |
| 11. Yes | 11. Tak | 11. Sie |
| 12. No | 12. Nie | 12. No |
| 13. I am disabled | 13. Ja jestem invalida | 13. Non capisco/ Sono handicappato |
| 14. I would like to buy | 14. Ile to kostujeza | 14. Lo prendo |
| 15. The menu, please | 15. Czy sa obiady? | 15. Posso vedere il menu? |
| 16. The bill, please | 16. Prosze o rachunek? | 16. Il conto, per favore? |
| 17. Police station | 17. Posterunek milicji | 17. La polizia |
| 18. What time is it? | 18. ktora jest godzina | 18. Che ore sono? |
| 19. Ladies | 19. Pani | 19. Signore |
| 20. Gentlemen | 20. panu | 20. Signori |

| ENGLISH | DUTCH-FLEMISH | SPANISH |
|---|---|---|
| 1. Good Morning | 1. Dag | 1. Buenos dias |
| 2. Good Evening | 2. Goeden Avond | 2. Buenas noches |
| 3. Goodbye | 3. Tot ziens | 3. Adios |
| 4. How much does this cost? | 4. Hoeveel | 4. ¿Cuanto cuesta esto? |
| 5. Many thanks | 5. Dank u zeer | 5. Muchas gracias |
| 6. I am ill | 6. ill | 6. Estoy enfermo |
| 7. I want a doctor | 7. Kunt u mij dichtst bijzijnde wijzen de dokter | 7. Llame a un medico |
| 8. Where is the bathroom? | 8. badkamer | 8. ¿Cuarto de baño? |
| 9. Please | 9. Alstublieft | 9. Por favor |
| 10. Ambulance | 10. Ambulance | 10. Ambulancia |
| 11. Yes | 11. Ja | 11. Si |
| 12. No | 12. Neen | 12. No |
| 13. I am disabled | 13. Ik hebeen gehandicapte | 13. Estoy invalido |
| 14. I would like to buy | 14. Wo kann ich | 14. Quiero comprar |
| 15. The menu, please | 15. Mag ik het menu zien? | 15. ¿El menu, por favor? |
| 16. The bill, please | 16. Mag ik de rekening, alstublieft? | 16. ¿La cuenta, por favor? |
| 17. Police station | 17. Kunt U mij dichst bujzijnde wilzen het politiebureau | 17. Llame a la policia |
| 18. What time is it? | 18. Hoe laat is het | 18. ¿Que hora es? |
| 19. Ladies | 19. Dames | 19. Senoras |
| 20. Gentlemen | 20. Heren | 20. Caballeros |

| ENGLISH | HEBREW |
|---|---|
| 1. Good Morning | 1. Boker tov |
| 2. Good Evening | 2. Erev tov |
| 3. Goodbye | 3. Shalom |
| 4. How much does this cost? | 4. Kama ze ole? |
| 5. Many Thanks | 5. Toda raba |
| 6. I am ill | 6. Ani chola |
| 7. I want a doctor | 7. Ani roset rofe |
| 8. Where is the bathroom | 8. Eifo ha ambatya |
| 9. Please | 9. B'vakasha |
| 10. Ambulance | 10. ambulance |
| 11. Yes | 11. Ken |
| 12. No | 12. Lo |
| 13. I am disabled | 13. Yeshli mum |
| 14. I would like to buy | 14. Ani rotse liknot |
| 15. The menu, please | 15. ha 'tafrit b'vakasha |
| 16. The bill, please | 16. Ha'heshbon b'vakasha |
| 17. Police station | 17. Tahanat Ha'mishtara |
| 18. What time is it? | 18. Ma hasha a? |
| 19. Ladies | 19. G'varotte |
| 20. Gentlemen | 20. G'varim |

# BIBLIOGRAPHY

*Access Amtrak,* Addison, Illinois: Amtrak Distribution Center.

*Access Travel—Airports Guide to Accessibility of Terminals,* Washington, D.C.: Access America.

Annand, Douglas. *The Wheelchair Traveler,* Milford, New Hampshire.

*Architectural Barriers Guide,* Chicago, Illinois: National Easter Seal Society.

Baxel, Eleanor Adams. *A Guide for the Solo Traveler Abroad,* Stockbridge, Massachusetts: Berkshire Traveler Press, 1979.

*Berlitz European Phrasebook 1984,* New York, New York: MacMillan Publishing Co., 1984.

Bowe, Frank. *Handicapped America—Barriers to Disabled People,* Harper & Row, 1978.

Davick, Alan, M.D., *First Travel—*Meds Timoniam, Maryland: Corporations of America, 1986.

Deak-Perera. *Getting Around Overseas: A Vacationer's Guide, Europe.*

*Dialysis Worldwide for the Traveling Patient,* Great Neck, New York: National Association of Patients on Hemodialysis and Transplantation.

Dupont, Herbert L., M.D. and Margaret W. Dupont. *Travel With Health,* New York, New York: Appleton-Century Crofts, 1981.

*Europe, 1980,* Stephen Birnbaum, ed., Boston, Massachusetts: Houghton-Mifflin Co., 1979.

Fielding, Temple. *Fielding's Europe, 1979,* New York, New York: William Morrow and Company, 1979.

*Fodor's Europe 1984,* New York, New York: Eugene Fodor, 1984.

*Fodor's South America 1984,* New York, New York: Eugene Fodor, 1984.

Grimes, Paul. "Practical Traveler: If Illness Strikes One Far From Home," *The New York Times,* New York, New York: The New York Times, January 1982.

*Guidelines for Developing Access Guides,* Albany, New York: New York State Easter Seal Society, 1979.

Hale, Glorya. *The Source Book for the Disabled,* New York, New York; London, England: Paddings Press Ltd., 1979.

Hughes, Charles A. *French Phrasebook and Dictionary,* New York, New York: Grosset and Dunlap, Inc., 1976.

*Information for Handicapped Travelers,* Washington, D.C.: National Library Service for the Blind and Physically Handicapped, Library of Congress, 1979.

Massow, Rosalind. *Now It's Your Turn to Travel,* MacMillan Publishing Co., 1970.

McNeil, Ian. *Disabled Travelers' International Phrasebook,* Milton Keynes, England: Disability Press, 1979.

Millery, Saul. *Super Traveler,* New York, New York: Holt, Rhinehart and Winston, 1980.

Peek, Ralph. *1984 TWA-Getaway Guide to Athens,* New York, New York: Simon and Schuster, Inc., 1984.

Rehabilitation and Research Training Center. *Travel for the Patient with Chronic Obstructive Pulmonary Disease,* Washington, D.C.: George Washington University Medical Center.

*The World Almanac and Book of Facts—1984,* New York, New York: Jane Flatt, 1984.

*Tips on Dealing With Deaf Passengers,* Washington, D.C.: Office of Alumni/Public Relations, Gallaudet College.

United States Customs Service. *Know Before You Go,* Publication Number 512, Washington, D.C., U.S. Customs Service, Department of the Treasury, 1983.

# INDEX

French West Indies
  tourist card and, 24
Fruits
  fresh, 48

Games, 35
Gasoline, 69
Germany, 65
"Green Card," 69
Greyhound bus, 65–66
Guam
  passport and, 24
Guatemala
  tourist card and, 24
Guidebooks, 22

Haggling, 81
Hairdressers, 76
Haiti
  tourist card and, 24
Hampton Court, England, 16
Handicapped Drivers Mobility Guide, 68
Hawaii, 78
  provisions for disabled in, 18
Health
  maintaining, 43–52
  problems, 90–91
Health insurance, 49
  additional, 90–91
Hearing aid batteries, 45
Home, protection of, 86–87
Home alarm system, 86–87
Hotel
  checking out of, 75–76
  concierge, 74
  libraries, 75
  lobbies, 75
  problems with, 91–92
  proceed directly to, 73
Hotels/motels
  with accessbile units in U.S., 153
Hyde Park, London, 78
Hydro-cortisone, 45

Ice cubes, 47
Immersion heater coil, 36
Immunizations, 43
Imports, restricted, 28
Information
  collection of, 16–20
  sources of, 16–17
Insect repellent, 45
Insulin, 46

Insulin reaction, 47
Insurance, 41–42
Interests, 15
Intermedic, 47
International Association of Medical
  Assistance to Travelers (IAMAT), 47
International Driving Permit, 69
Israel, 78
Italy, 13
Itinerary, copy of, 87

Jamaica
  tourist card and, 24
Jet lag, 73
Jewelry, 32

Language differences, 76–77
Languages.
  See also Dictionaries;
    Foreign phrase vocabulary cards
Languages, foreign, 15
Laundry kit, 36
Laxatives, 44
Limosines, 73
London, England, 13, 78
Luggage
  restrictions on, 33–34

Mail, 40–41, 86
Maps, 67
Meal times, 77
Meal voucher, 88
Medic Alert, 46
Medic Alert Foundation, 46
Medical assistance, 6, 154–155
Medical documents, 44
Medications, 44
  See also Drug interactions; Insulin;
    Insulin reactions
Metric conversion tables, 128
Mexico
  tourist card and, 24
Michelin Guidebooks, 22
Money, 28–30
  bank transfer, 94
  cash, 29–30
  credit cards, 94–95
  exchange of, 75
  running out of, 94
  travelers checks, 29, 92
Motion sickness medication, 45

Nap, 4, 44